Mastering Cycling

John Howard

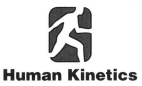

Human Kinetics

Library of Congress Cataloging-in-Publication Data

Howard, John, 1947-
 Mastering cycling / John Howard.
   p. cm. -- (The master athlete series)
 ISBN-13: 978-0-7360-8677-6 (soft cover)
 ISBN-10: 0-7360-8677-3 (soft cover)
 1. Cycling--Training. I. Title.
 GV1048.H68 2010
 796.6--dc22

                          2010011345

ISBN-10: 0-7360-8677-3 (print)
ISBN-13: 978-0-7360-8677-6 (print)

Copyright © 2010 by Human Kinetics, Inc.

This publication is written and published to provide accurate and authoritative information relevant to the subject matter presented. It is published and sold with the understanding that the author and publisher are not engaged in rendering legal, medical, or other professional services by reason of their authorship or publication of this work. If medical or other expert assistance is required, the services of a competent professional person should be sought.

The Web addresses cited in this text were current as of April 2010, unless otherwise noted.

Acquisitions Editor; Tom Heine; **Developmental Editor:** Laura Floch; **Assistant Editor:** Elizabeth Evans; **Copyeditor:** Joy Wotherspoon; **Permission Manager:** Martha Gullo; **Graphic Designer:** Joe Buck; **Graphic Artist:** Tara Welsch; **Cover Designer:** Keith Blomberg; **Photographer (cover):** Scott McDermott/Aurora Photos; **Photographer (interior):** Neil Bernstein, unless otherwise noted; **Visual Production Assistant:** Joyce Brumfield; **Photo Production Manager:** Jason Allen; **Art Manager and Illustrator:** Kelly Hendren; **Associate Art Manager:** Alan L. Wilborn; **Printer:** Sheridan Books

Human Kinetics books are available at special discounts for bulk purchase. Special editions or book excerpts can also be created to specification. For details, contact the Special Sales Manager at Human Kinetics.

Printed in the United States of America   10 9 8 7 6 5 4 3 2 1

The paper in this book is certified under a sustainable forestry program.

Human Kinetics
Web site: www.HumanKinetics.com

United States: Human Kinetics
P.O. Box 5076
Champaign, IL 61825-5076
800-747-4457
e-mail: humank@hkusa.com

Canada: Human Kinetics
475 Devonshire Road Unit 100
Windsor, ON N8Y 2L5
800-465-7301 (in Canada only)
e-mail: info@hkcanada.com

Europe: Human Kinetics
107 Bradford Road
Stanningley
Leeds LS28 6AT, United Kingdom
+44 (0) 113 255 5665
e-mail: hk@hkeurope.com

Australia: Human Kinetics
57A Price Avenue
Lower Mitcham, South Australia 5062
08 8372 0999
e-mail: info@hkaustralia.com

New Zealand: Human Kinetics
P.O. Box 80
Torrens Park, South Australia 5062
0800 222 062
e-mail: info@hknewzealand.com

E4942

In memory of Bill Edwards.
He was the spark that lit my coaching career.

Contents

Foreword

John Howard is one of those special people who can be classified as a pioneer among the field of outstanding American cyclists. Revered among fellow U.S. Bicycling Hall of Famers, John has been on the forefront of innovation on the American and world cycling scene for most of his life. He has never been afraid to try out new ideas, to identify and embrace unique challenges, or to think outside the box.

Ever since his beginnings in Springfield, Missouri, John Howard has been a man ahead of his time. This can be both a blessing and a source of frustration because the process of getting others to understand and accept new concepts can take a long time. John has developed many ideas for training, racing, and nutrition, including his unique bike-fitting protocol. However, it has often taken some time for the American cycling community to accept the product of his genius. Always the perfect gentleman, he never gives up moving forward, and that is the sign of a true winner.

Part of being a pioneer in sport is being able to sort out the good ideas from the garbage. Over the past 60 years, a lot of bad science has been published in the cycling literature. John's judgment in weeding out the good from the bad has been superb. For example, physiology pundits used to believe that after the age of 30, a person's athletic performance would begin to steadily decline, and there was nothing that could be done about it. Obviously, John never accepted this pronouncement, and he simply continued to achieve new personal records and set new absolute records. It has since been proven repeatedly that an athlete's performance does not have to deteriorate if certain key adjustments are made to the training protocol. It now is widely accepted that we don't just get older; we can continue to get better with age. All it takes is attention to details such as those that are presented in this book.

At age 62, John continues to maintain an extremely high level of fitness, and he remains on the cutting edge of training technology. UCLA basketball coach John Wooden, one of the greatest coaches of all time, defined success as peace of mind, which is the result of knowing in your heart that you have done everything possible to become the very best that you are capable of becoming. John Howard is one of those men who definitely meets John Wooden's criterion for success. He is one of the finest, most accomplished, and most humble gentlemen in the sport.

John's feats as a sportsman are legendary: three-time Olympian, four-time U.S. national road race champion, gold medalist in the Pan American Games, 24-hour world record holder (593 miles), second-place finisher in the inaugural

Race Across America (RAAM), Hawaiian Ironman champion, holder of the land-speed record on a bicycle (over 152 mph), and much more. What is truly amazing is the broad range of his cycling achievements.

John's new PowerFitte bike-fitting technology is just the most recent example of his position at the forefront of new techniques for the cycling community. His systematic protocol has made many of his clients more powerful, more comfortable, faster, and happier on their bikes.

Fortunately for the cycling community, and most especially for the masters cycling community, John has assembled all of his experience and wisdom into this book. Many of the training methods that are aimed at improving the performance of masters cyclists appear nowhere else in the coaching literature.

Bill Edwards, PhD
www.PerformanceEdge-R.com

Preface

Albert Einstein once said, "There are only two ways to live your life. One is as though nothing is a miracle. The other is as though everything is a miracle." I vastly prefer the latter to the former. Life in itself is a miracle, and I have found cycling to be a great way to enjoy the many miracles of living life on this planet. Ever since I first discovered cycling, I have loved feeling my heart pumping energy into my limbs and covering mile after mile by my own power. I began by pedaling through the beautiful Ozark Mountains and rural countryside near Springfield, Missouri, and now I frequent the sunlit coastal beauty of southern California.

I have had a lifelong love affair with the bicycle. In spite of my interest in fast machines and my desire to ride bikes with the latest technology in frames and components, I maintain a deep appreciation for bikes of all ages. I like to ride on bikes that were built 50 to 60 years ago when milk was delivered to your door by men in starched white uniforms. Those relics of the past recall simpler times, when bikes crafted from steel by artisans were thought to be as light as spiders. However, as Lance Armstrong titled his book, it's not about the bike; any bike will do. For me, it's about feeling the joy of being alive and living life to its fullest.

Some of us ride to save money, some want to lose weight, and others want to define themselves in competition with displays of hard-earned athleticism. Some cycle to deny their advancing years. Whatever the reason for training, riding, and competing, age is the great equalizer. Enthusiasm for the sport is a positive attribute, but I can't help but wonder how Lance Armstrong will deal with the inevitable onset of years. Although their hearts were still passionately involved with the sport, Greg LeMond and others before him have had to confront the issues of aging.

I have gone from being the big dog on the block to matching strokes with professionals who are 35 years younger. At times, this has made me hit the wall. Recently, I was climbing a hill on Del Dios Highway above Lake Hodges in northern San Diego County. While pressing the flesh and reaching deep for the reserve of energy that had seldom failed me, I realized in a single, gasping, heart-governed instant that I wasn't going to find it this time. I was forced to forget the pace I had desired to maintain and to find a level of effort that my body could accommodate. It was then that I remembered why I ride in the first place: for the love of the experience. Love it! This sport is about life, *yours!*

Acknowledgments

I would like to thank Rene Maurer for her tireless contributions to clarify my well-meaning, but often times disconnected, thoughts. Without Rene, *Mastering Cycling* simply could not have been written, so the first toast to the success of this book is to her. Many thanks to Laura Floch for her invaluable suggestions and patience during the editing process. I would also like to give credit to FiTTE co-founder, Dr. Ernie Ferrel, whose knowledge of human anatomy and his clarification of how muscles work on the bike was essential. I also want to thank the C.H.E.K. Institute, Paul Chek, and Chris Mound for setting me on the correct course for cycling-related flexibility and strength training. Thanks to all the cyclists I interviewed and those who contributed photographs, as well as the models who dedicated their time and energy, all of whom helped us capture the spirit of this book.

Credits

© John Howard Collection. Pages 2, 4, 17, 25, 27

© Jerry Murray. Page 3

Photo by Albert C. Gross, copyright 2010. Page 7

Courtesy of The Bicycle Museum of America/New Bremen, Ohio. Page 8

© Kathy Taylor/Link Lindquist. Page 19

© Toshio Okano - iDigitalPix. Pages 24, 137

© Harry Howard. Page 26

Jerry Landrum/BMXmania.com. Page 28

© Tom Moran. Page 47

© Anne Cram Designs. Page 82

© Victor Copeland. Page 92

Property of John A. Sinibaldi. Page 112

© Mike Gladu/Velodrome.com. Page 125

© Bryan Van Vleet. Page 135

© Hillard Salas. Page 156

Courtesy of www.1888scanvan.com. Page 161

Introduction

USA Cycling, the organization that governs bicycle racing in America, defines a Masters cyclist as thirty and older. In terms of participation, this means that racing in the U.S. is essentially a master's sport. Whether you are a competitive or recreational cyclist, I want your passion for riding bicycles to preserve your life's balance. This book will explore cycling as a body-friendly exercise that can enhance the substance and improve the longevity of your life. As a masters cyclist, I view the aging process as a personal challenge to recreate a broader variety of techniques that contribute to a healthy lifestyle. It doesn't matter if you are a spin-class aficionado, a weekend warrior, or a seasoned competitor; I am committed to helping you scale the rungs of the cycling performance ladder.

You will learn how the sport can help you sort out the priorities of work and family commitments and relieve the associated stress. My approach is to use the bike as both a reward for a job well done and as a stimulus to fire the momentum that drives your life. This mind/body stimulation is a critical, but often forgotten, element of exercise. The beauty of cycling is that it blends a utilitarian element to this self-improvement formula. *Mastering Cycling* will increase your efficiency on and off the bike, regardless of your age or level of experience.

Power, comfort, and safety are the components that I consider to be priorities for an enjoyable cycling experience. I will explain the mechanical and biomechanical elements of an effective setup that can be tailored to your individual requirements. I will tell you how to increase your flexibility and strengthen the primary support muscles of the knees and core, accompanied by an array of photographs that illustrate the correct form. Another component that is needed to build an efficient power base is the improvement of pedaling efficiency. I use a variety of old and new technologies to improve your skill level in order to get you up to speed and on the road. As I have done with amateurs and pros alike, I will explain how you can greatly improve your bike handling skills to gain more confidence while riding in the pack and in traffic.

In my mind, the term "training" really means "playing," and the actual process is broken out into blocks of play. The performance concepts explained here are innovative, and you may find that my priorities differ from those of other coaches. These ideas represent the views of several respected coaches who specialize in masters cyclists. These principles are the basis of our collective wisdom, illustrated and supported by interviews with some of the multiple world champions we have coached. The competitive ground in cycling is as fertile as any sport on the planet, and bike choices reflect this diversity. I will discuss the types of bikes available that can enhance your enjoyment of this specialty-driven sport.

I will also delve into the menagerie of competitive and non-competitive events available to masters. We will look at the strategies associated with each type of race and the sport-specific training for each. I will also cover injuries and age-related issues that masters cyclists typically encounter. Masters cyclists are not "over the hill." Regardless of their ages, they ride "over the hill," again and again, finding fun events in which to participate and races in which to compete. They also find comradery and lasting friendships as they ride the roads and trails to better fitness, health, and enjoyment.

The Masters Cyclist

started riding seriously after reading *The Big Loop*, a 1955 novel by Claire Huchet Bishop. It was about a French boy, Andre, who beat incredible odds to achieve his dream of racing in the Tour de France. The wonderful pencil sketches of the riders with their spare tires slung about their shoulders really captured my imagination and inspired me to be a cyclist.

My first serious bike was a Schwinn Continental. I rode it hard for several years until I was T-boned by a car pulling out of a local drive-in restaurant. I upgraded to a Schwinn Sierra with a triple-chain ring. Before my first race, at age 19, I purchased the flagship of the Schwinn line, a $195 state-of-the-art Paramount. The 1966 event was a 105-mile (169 km) road race, and I rode that canary-yellow bike to a gold medal in the 1971 Pan American Games in Cali, Colombia.

Remember the defining events that knit together the fabric of your cycling experience: your first bike, your first significant ride, the first big terrain hurdle you conquered, and many other nostalgic details. A pleasurable bike ride or a particularly satisfying race gives you the desire to get back out there and recapture that experience. As you grow older, your specific cycling goals may change, but the general desire to feel good persists. Whether you are a serious racer, an endurance athlete, or a weekend cruiser, continue to ride as long as cycling satisfies whatever desire it creates in you.

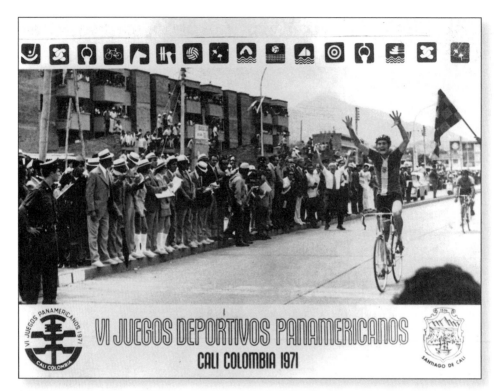

John Howard winning the 1971 Pan American road race in Cali, Colombia.

WHO ARE MASTERS CYCLISTS?

Masters cyclists do not adhere to a textbook definition—they come from diverse backgrounds and in all shapes, sizes, and ages. Categories for racing depend on the promoters or sponsors, but generally, masters cyclists are men and women over the age of 30 who have a passion for cycling. Some are former professional or amateur cyclists who raced; others never seriously rode a bicycle until they were in their 30s, 40s, or older. They can be young adults with or without families, middle-aged enthusiasts, retirees, or grandparents. They can be teachers, mechanics, or neurosurgeons. Some enjoy weekend jaunts, and others ride 100 miles (161 km) or more per week. Some tour across a nation on their bicycles, while others simply ride to have breakfast with friends. Some are professional cyclists, and others are novices in the sport. They all share one commonality: They love to ride.

As a cycling and multisport coach, I most commonly see recreational enthusiasts who begin their training with the caveat that they are not athletes and have no desire to compete. After developing their cycling skills and receiving encouragement from their peers, they often become competitive. With proper training and effective conditioning, focused athletes can be as powerful in their

Jerry and Sarah

My friend Jerry has been cycling since he was a teenager. For most of his 72 years, he has lived to ride his bike. Jerry raced bicycles in the late 1950s, when the U.S. Cycling Federation was known as the Amateur Bicycle League of America. During those days, cycling was a little-known, subcultural activity. Jerry was also a successful middle-distance runner who played mean games of tennis, handball, and tournament pool. While raising his children, he regarded cycling as fresh-air and blue-sky therapy, but as he grew older, his competitive spirit began to reemerge. Jerry attended our San Diego racing camp in 1997, and bicycle racing became his compulsion once again.

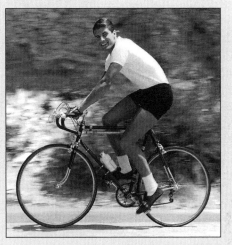

Jerry Murray on his steel racer in 1957.

Recently, Jerry told me that after more than half a century of cycling with only a few minor mishaps, he had missed the last step while walking down the stairs to his basement. That misstep cost Jerry his mobility and freedom. Just after having surgery to repair severely damaged quadriceps, he asked for my counsel. Regaining his physical health and taking his body to a higher level of cycling fitness are Jerry's fervent goals.

Sarah, another friend of mine, is 42, a wife, the mother of a toddler, a university professor, and the most humble and accomplished amateur athlete I know. She practices yoga and both downhill and cross-country skiing. She is also a high-ranking age-group Ironman triathlete, and

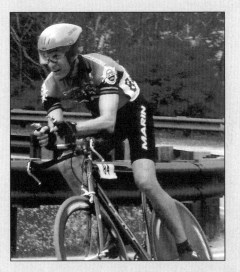

Jerry Murray at the national championships in 2007 on a carbon-fiber bike.

was the overall female winner of the 2007 Carlsbad Marathon. Sarah's model on balancing the essential elements of training with a busy life is a valuable lesson in time management.

40s and 50s as in their teens and 20s. Most masters would agree that cycling is a sport for life since it offers so many opportunities for self-discovery, healthful longevity, and raising environmental consciousness.

WHY CYCLING?

The sport of masters cycling is growing quickly. In *Masters Cycling*, JoAnne Klimovich Harrop says that masters cyclists are now more secure financially, more able to travel to nonlocal cycling events, and more interested in staying physically fit. Cycling gives them the opportunity to train or simply to ride with their spouses or friends. Aging cyclists can celebrate landmark birthdays by competing in a race or completing an endurance ride. The National Off-Road Biking Association (NORBA) and the United States Cycling Federation (USCF) enjoyed a combined membership increase of 8 percent for cyclists aged 35 and older between July 2005 and June 2006. Cyclists between the ages of 35 and 44 make up the largest contingent in both organizations at 33 percent and 36 percent, respectively. *Cycling South Australia*, a Web site for competitive masters cyclists, states that masters cyclists represent the strongest segment of growth in cycling across the country "down under." Masters cycling organizations have popped up in many countries all over the globe for recreational riders and serious competitors.

I am impressed by the homemakers, the corporate warriors who work 40 to 60 hours per week, and the busy professionals who never ventured into anything athletic before discovering cycling. Many masters are empty nesters hoping to reclaim their youthful vigor (and physiques) and look to cycling as a new frontier. I am gratified by the steady flow of people I have had the privilege of advising over the years. They discover or rediscover cycling for a variety of reasons, and many come to the sport in their later years. Ultimately, the reasons for becoming a masters cyclist are as diverse as the personalities and histories of the participants.

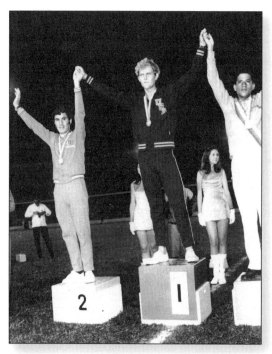

John Howard on the podium in Cali, Colombia, 1971.

In the United States, there are more cyclists than skiers, golfers, and tennis players combined. According to a 2008 survey that was conducted by the National Sporting Goods Association (NSGA), 54.9 million people ride bicycles as a regular form of exercise. Many love cycling because of the way it feels to take a fast descent down a winding, tree-lined road with the wind in their faces. Others love the satisfaction of reaching the summit of a challenging climb. Riding a bike is all about discovering who you are and how far or fast you can go under your own power. Some cyclists are equipment junkies who pride themselves in having the latest and coolest gear. Others couldn't care less about the mechanical aspects of the sport, preferring the experience of the ride, becoming more fit, and the opportunity for social interaction.

Cycling and Personal Enjoyment

The social atmosphere of cycling has changed since the early 1960s. Riding a bike to junior high or high school in those days was a very uncool activity. A classmate told me, "You drive or walk, period. You don't ride that iron mistress, especially to school." I like the term *iron mistress* although it no longer applies to modern bikes, which are often constructed from aluminum, carbon fiber, and titanium. At the time, bikes were sold in toy stores, and mom-and-pop bike shops sold them along with lawn mowers. Cycling was a kid's activity, something few self-respecting grown-ups would do.

I went to college in the '70s, when the social atmosphere concerning cycling was changing to one of cautious acceptability as physical fitness and cycling became synonymous. Those of us who rode were still a minority, and in my conservative Midwestern community, cycling was still considered weird. Regardless of the social ramifications, I was obsessed with cycling. Through my efforts in the saddle, I developed a strong aerobic power base that helped me with other sports, such as swimming and running. Obsession can be a valuable component of success, along with a healthy helping of confidence.

Although obsession has given way to moderation as the years have passed, I'm still commuting on a bike after more than 40 years. I ride for the joy and therapy of cycling. I view cycling as part of my disposition, character, and creed.

Today, social opportunities for cyclists are abundant. Cycling clubs, which are plentiful, usually offer groups with various levels of ability and experience. Some cyclists embark on serious rides that last three hours or more. Others travel at a leisurely pace to their favorite restaurants or coffee shops for breakfast. Long-time friendships and even marriages have resulted from club associations. Web sites and forums exist where cyclists can meet to discuss pertinent topics, share experiences, or announce organized rides. Cyclists from all over the country can arrange to meet at an event and ride together. The possibilities are limitless.

Cycling and Physical Fitness

Cycling is a stable, low-impact exercise that increases joint mobility and stability. The cyclical motion nurtures the joint cartilage and strengthens the surrounding musculature, decreasing the odds of subsequent injury. However, riding bicycles, whether stationary or mobile, that are not properly fitted can lead to injuries. The bicycle is an effective tool for recovery when used correctly.

Many of my masters clients share a rich athletic history, most often in running or swimming. Recently, I have seen former golfers and tennis players turn to cycling after abandoning their sport because of chronic overuse injuries. Some athletes are former team-sport participants who cut their teeth on baseball, basketball, or football. I'm intrigued by the fact that more of my contemporaries are gravitating toward cycling. Complaints of debilitating knee, back, and hip injuries have brought many masters athletes to the sport. Others are looking for more adventure in their workouts. Whatever attracts athletes from other sports, I think the appeal of open-road adventure is a big part of the equation.

As any older distance runner will tell you, running is not kind to joints, muscles, and ligaments. Many masters runners have gravitated toward cycling because it's easier on their bodies, and they enjoy covering more ground under their own power. A masters runner who can cover 20 miles (32 km) in less than four hours can ride 60 miles (97 km) or more in the same time with minimal training in the saddle. My occasional running buddy Ted began accompanying me on a few of my rare century (100-mile) rides. His thoughts are worth heeding: "I never thought of myself as much of a cyclist, but the joints certainly appreciate the break, and my cardio levels are now about the same on the bike as when I do my hard runs." Ted is a small-boned masters runner and cyclist who, at 60 years of age, still uses track running for the majority of his training. A look at the membership ranks of ultradistance cyclists reveals a fair number of former runners who now cycle exclusively for exercise.

Older swimmers, many of whom still enjoy pool workouts and open-water swims, are adding cycling to their workouts. Some are budding triathletes, and others are excited about riding in wide-open spaces. Swimmers bring a wonderful sense of discipline to their cycling. Most of the masters swimmers I have coached have no difficulty following regimented programs since they have done this in the pool most of their lives with metronomic regularity.

Former president George W. Bush is one of the statistics. Like many runners who have punished their knees for 30 years or more, our former chief executive was advised by his doctors to try biking. According to his media advisor and frequent cycling companion, Mark McKinnon, Bush became a "biking maniac." During his presidency, he spent many hours riding his carbon-fiber Trek mountain bike in and around the DC area, as well as on his ranch in Crawford, Texas. "He's obsessed with it," McKinnon said. "He now likes to do nothing but work out on his bike, and he does it with a frenzy that is reserved for people like Lance Armstrong."

Most of the masters athletes participate in more than one form of cycling. The equipment has many manifestations, including mountain bikes, single-speed or track bikes, hybrids, which combine features from mountain and road bikes for greater stability and comfort, tandems, custom three-wheelers, recumbents, and pedaled watercraft. Each has its own appeal. Cycling, regardless of its form, is the primary panacea for masters athletes. Repetitive motion and traumatic injuries are so common in collegiate sports that few masters play tackle football or rugby. If you check the average age of the participants in any of the hundreds of charity rides or punishing ultradistance events, such as the Race Across AMerica (RAAM) and the Ironman Triathlon, you will find plenty of highly competitive masters celebrating their fitness.

Cycling and Competitive Goals

In the late 1970s, my coach kicked me off the U.S. national cycling team because I was too old. During my military days, my drill sergeant said that the Chinese used the same symbol for both crisis and opportunity. "Crisis," he used to tell us, "is an opportunity riding the dangerous winds." Although I did not appreciate being expelled from the cycling team, I eventually realized that my coach had done me a favor. His actions motivated me to readjust my priorities and begin my triathlon career.

When I could no longer race with the national team, I trained for the Ironman Triathlon in Hawaii. Ironman was a full-time job for more than two years that required me to supplement my earlier training in swimming and running. I won the overall championship on my second try in 1981. I went on to train for the Race Across America, which in its inaugural year was called The Great American Bike Race. This goal proved to be unrealistic because I needed to sleep in order to perform. Sometimes we must rethink goals that are ill-conceived, but this process is part of the journey to self-discovery. My second-place finish in the RAAM led me to attempt the 24-hour world distance record, which I

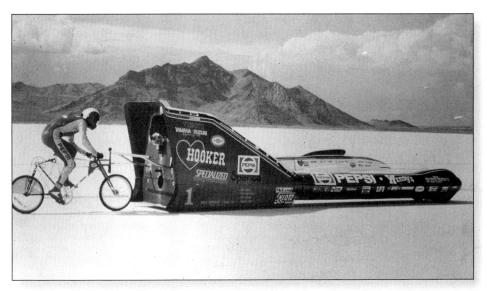

John Howard on the Bonneville Salt Flats in Utah in 1985, setting a world speed record at 152.2 mph (245 kph).

grabbed in 1987 with a hard 539-mile (867 km) ride. This discovery process and the accompanying training consumed three years of my life. The last part of my reinvention involved a three-year attempt to break the world land-speed record on the Bonneville Salt Flats in Utah.

This particular record began in 1897 when Charlie "Mile-a-Minute" Murphy was paced by a Long Island express train at 60 miles (97 km) per hour. The record was broken numerous times over the next three quarters of a century, culminating with Dr. Al Abbott's 140-mph (225 kph) ride on the Bonneville Salt Flats in 1973. Breaking that record was a dream I'd had since the age of 12 after reading an advertising comic about French six-day bike-racing star, Alf Letourner. In 1941, the "Red Devil" set a new world land-speed record of 108.92 mph (175 kph) in Bakersfield, California while being paced by a quarter-midget racecar. My crew and I went through some dangerous and exhilarating experiences, first at Bonneville, then in Mexico, before returning to Bonneville to claim the record at 152.2 mph (245 kph).

If circumstances force you to give up a sport, look at it as an opportunity for personal growth. If traffic makes you afraid to brave the mean streets of the city, try mountain biking on trails where motor vehicles are not permitted. Perhaps you long to be an ultradistance athlete, but you consistently drop out during long training rides. Consider other areas where your talents might lie. For example, Teresa, who was in her late thirties and newly divorced, decided to train for an Ironman triathlon and had poor results. It became apparent that she was more of a sprinter than an endurance athlete, so she turned to match sprints and 1-kilometer time trials at a local velodrome.

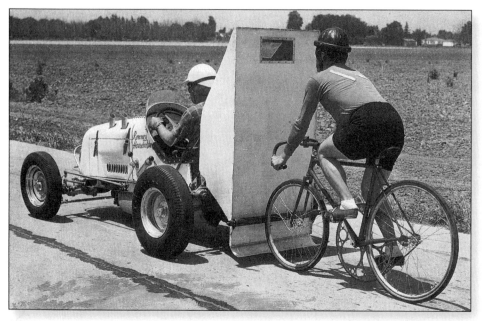

Alf LeTourner, the Red Devil, setting the world speed record at 109 mph (175 kph) in Bakersfield, California in 1941.

I'm a professional cycling and triathlon coach, and during my long tenure, I have observed common physiological issues that keep masters cyclists from realizing their full potential. These issues must be addressed in order to help their bodies properly adapt to the sport of cycling. These same weaknesses also make masters athletes more prone to injury. Cycling offers many cardio-respiratory and cardiovascular benefits; however, most masters cyclists have very tight extremities, and many neglect their upper bodies. Balanced training for strength and flexibility seems to be missing from the training programs of both younger and older masters, including those cycling for the first time and serious competitive masters racers, who may be unaware of the limiting effect of hours in the saddle with poorly balanced musculature.

Having coached hundreds of competitive masters cyclists to more than 140 national titles, I have had to keep my clients from doing too much too soon. Many of my best athletes look enviously at the inflated training schedules of 25-year-old, full-time professional racers and think that such a plan will work for them. This is a huge mistake. Masters who follow a diverse plan of cross-training and sensible mileage will ultimately experience greater success and fewer injuries. In my experience, this is a tough lesson for most type-A masters to learn. I have found that masters cyclists who have discretionary income and interests outside of cycling are the ones who end up on the three-tiered podium.

Anyone who has experienced the rigors of child rearing or corporate maneuvering knows the importance of setting goals. Most goal-conscious masters have a passion for training and racing, and define their goals by what inspires them. Your goal may be to ride a century on your 50th birthday, save money by riding to work three times per week, compete in your first bike race, spend the summer with your spouse or friends cycling across the country, or conquer a local mountain on your bike. Whatever your dreams are, set realistic goals to achieve them. These experiences become the motivators that move your life along the path to satisfaction and fulfillment.

Same Sport, New Challenges

Masters cyclists face a different set of challenges than juniors, pros, and younger amateur cyclists do. They have more responsibilities and less time to train, and age-related physical problems begin to emerge. This chapter discusses the important aspects of cycling that will help you enjoy the experience without suffering from time-consuming mistakes.

In my nearly 50 years as a cyclist, I have progressively accumulated knowledge. My objective is to provide information that will prevent frustration, refine your techniques, and enhance your cycling experience. I want to temper your understanding with an appreciation for what the bicycle can do for you, help you celebrate the gift of life, and give you an aesthetic awareness of the world around you.

Like aikido, a lifelong martial art in which masters do not hit their prime until they are in their 80s, knowledge of cycling develops over time. This sport can be yours for life. Cycling is an enjoyable pastime that offers opportunities for social interaction and many health advantages. However, in our busy world, squeezing another activity into an already full schedule can be difficult. We must also acknowledge and address issues associated with aging.

BENEFITS OF CYCLING

As we age, we experience a decline in cardiorespiratory function, strength, flexibility, and balance. It also takes us longer to recover from injuries. Fortunately, cycling is an ideal practice for postponing the inevitable ravages of aging. This wonderful, low-impact, aerobic activity contributes to cardiorespiratory health, keeps the joints well lubricated and the muscles strong, and relieves accumulated stress.

Increased Aerobic Capacity

I enjoy coaching age-group cyclists and multisport athletes. One of the most rewarding parts of the process is identifying and measuring the individual aspects of physical performance that have diminished, or likely will diminish, with age. I create a plan for each athlete to help counter the deterioration associated with aging and to improve performance with time. For example, the oxygen-carrying capacity of all athletes gradually diminishes with age. I saw a 17 percent drop in my own $\dot{V}O_2$max between my first test at age 20 and a test administered at age 58. Other masters cyclists who have tested themselves at similar ages confirm this finding. Hypothetically, this kind of loss signals the end of a career for an endurance athlete. Fortunately, the human body is an amazingly complex collection of systems, and oxygen transfer is just one measurement of its performance.

After you have achieved the weekly mileage totals you desire, you can maintain a high level of cardiorespiratory fitness with short aerobic workouts of about 15 minutes on the trainer, followed by 15 minutes of anaerobic intervals. The anaerobic efforts are very effective in maintaining your ability to process oxygen. Masters racers who follow this plan find their time trials are comparable to or faster than many racers in professional categories for the same distance. Once you have established your mileage base, I recommend reducing your hours and miles to focus more on recovery. A thorough coach will monitor an athlete's progress with basic physiological tests. Results of $\dot{V}O_2$max testing are not always the best indicator of performance for masters cyclists, or even for elite endurance athletes. More-thorough testing examines steady-state power output at the lactate threshold. The lactate threshold is the maximum effort that an athlete can maintain without an increase in blood lactate. Effort beyond that point will cause blood lactate, along with the high acid levels, to increase until the athlete is compelled to slow down or quit entirely. Lactate thresholds in elite masters racers have tested as high as 90 percent of $\dot{V}O_2$max.

Consider a 2008 study by the news staff of CTV, a Canadian television network, which found that aerobic activities, such as cycling, are especially important in the middle years of life. Declining aerobic capacity may be inevitable after middle age since most people lose about 5 milliliters per kilogram-minute every decade. Once the capacity falls below 18 milliliters per kilogram per minute for men and 15 milliliters per kilogram per minute for women, it becomes very difficult to do almost anything without experiencing severe fatigue. A typical 60-year-old, sedentary male has an aerobic capacity of about 25 milliliters per kilogram per minute; his aerobic capacity would have been twice that at age 20. Research studies have found that high-intensity aerobic exercise over a relatively long period of time can boost a masters athlete's aerobic capacity by 25 percent. For the 60-year-old sedentary male, that is equivalent to a gain of 6 milliliters per kilogram per minute. Imagine gaining 10 to 12 more years to spend riding your bike!

"There seems to be good evidence that the conservation of maximal oxygen intake increases the likelihood that the healthy elderly person will retain functional independence," said Dr. Roy Shephard, author of the study and faculty member of the University of Toronto's department of physical education and health and the department of public health sciences. Other benefits include reduced risk of serious disease, faster recovery after injury or illness, and decreased risk of falling due to lack of muscle strength, balance, and coordination.

Although that study touted high-intensity training for boosting aerobic capacity, an August 2007 study found that middle-aged people could obtain other health benefits from moderate exercise, such as reducing triglycerides in the blood. High triglyceride levels are linked to arterial disease and pancreatitis. Moderate exercise can also boost the amount of high-density lipoprotein (HDL), or good cholesterol, in the blood. Other studies praise the benefits of strength training for people in their 80s and those who have heart problems. In April 2007, a British study found that the 50-plus age group was more likely to exercise with their peers but would rather work out alone than among spandex-clad 20-somethings.

Increased Strength and Flexibility

Although the sport offers many aerobic and cardiorespiratory benefits, most masters cyclists are missing a few ingredients that should be addressed to improve their experience and to cement my promise that cycling is indeed a sport for life. A balance between flexibility and strength seems to be the main component missing for both younger and older masters, whether they are cycling for the first time or training for serious competitive races. Therefore, masters riders need to modify their training priorities, regardless of their abilities. For most masters, I reduce the hours in the saddle and use this additional time to increase flexibility and to balance muscle strength. Consequently, athletes gain a greater range of motion for critical joints and muscles, which improves their ability to leverage muscles and increase power output.

Peak power output can be an excellent indicator of performance level for all cycling disciplines. This approach is nontraditional, but I think it better addresses the needs of masters athletes. Cycling coaches have traditionally increased training volume to induce muscular overload and adaptation. This practice is especially inappropriate for masters, who typically recover more slowly due to a number of physiological factors. Reduced mileage and short-sprint training intervals lead to substantial gains in peak power output and maximal capacity. This type of workout also increases the $\dot{V}O_2$max as compared to workouts of lower intensity and longer duration.

Increased Bone Density

Varying the type and intensity of the exercises during workouts can also enhance bone health. Evidence exists that the risk of lower than normal bone density, or osteopenia, increases significantly for people who ride bicycles exclusively and avoid weight-bearing activities, such as running or weight training. Many people have abandoned high-impact activities because of fears that their joints or bones may be injured; however, weight-bearing workouts prompt the body to create more bone mass. Bones weaken and fracture more easily without applied stress, as illustrated by the rapid loss of bone density experienced by astronauts living in a weightless environment.

Ed Pavelka, who has been a friend of mine for nearly 40 years, publishes the weekly e-mail newsletter for the Web site www.RoadBikeRider.com. On his Web site, Ed featured Dr. Gabe Mirkin, who discussed the question of whether bicycling reduces bone density, increasing risk for fractures and osteoporosis. Dr. Mirkin claimed, "This is a myth that is not supported by any good data. A study from Manchester Metropolitan University in the UK shows that sprint cyclists have denser bones than long-distance cyclists, who have denser bones than the sedentary control subjects. While cyclists have less-dense bones than weight lifters and football players, they still have denser bones than long-distance cyclists, who have denser bones than people who do not exercise. The greater the force on bones during exercise, the denser the bones become. So any type of exercise is good for your bones, and a sedentary lifestyle is bad for bones" (*Medicine and Science in Sports and Exercise*, March 2009).

Sports physicians are seeing professional and amateur cyclists, including those in their late 20s and 30s who have raced or trained for 7 to 10 years, fracture their hips and femurs after seemingly innocuous falls. X-rays show evidence of below-normal bone densities. A different study published by Mirkin's journal compared the spines of competitive, male road cyclists with those of athletes of a similar age who actively pursued other forms of exercise. The bone-mineral density of the cyclists was significantly lower than that of the members of the control group. Osteopenia (lower than normal bone density) and osteoporosis (low bone density with increased risk for fractures) were more likely to occur for the cyclists, even though they were taking more calcium supplements than the members of the control group. Another study comparing road cyclists to mountain bikers found that the mountain bikers had greater bone density. The study attributed the results to the roughness of the terrain, which placed increased stress on the bones. Since the development of bone mass peaks in our late 20s, if young cyclists train exclusively on their bikes during those years, their bones, including their spines, will be more likely to fracture in a fall.

Cycling and Life-Threatening Illnesses

Although awareness of poor bone density in athletes is growing, it does not capture attention or induce fear the same way that a life-threatening illness does. We are all familiar with Lance Armstrong's well-documented recovery from cancer, his successfully resumed competitive career, and his tireless foundation work to fund both cancer research and public awareness of the disease. Plenty of research demonstrates that recovery from cancer treatment accelerates when patients participate in supervised training, and cycling is one of the most popular forms of exercise. Rehabilitative training focuses on developing an individualized exercise program to address the needs of the cancer patient while improving stamina, endurance, and joint mobility.

My friend Bill used cycling to salvage his former fitness during a two-year battle with non-Hodgkin's lymphoma. Brutal chemotherapy sessions and plummeting blood counts made walking up a flight of stairs nearly impossible. However, Bill timed his stationary-trainer workouts for the times of physical highs and spent the low points in recovery. When his tumors went into remission, Bill's immune system began to recover. His strength returned, and he celebrated his successful recovery with a series of victories in the Senior Olympics. Bill was in his 70s, and I find his achievements to be on par with Lance Armstrong's victories at the Tour de France after recovering from cancer. Bill's fight continued as he faced a new round of chemotherapy. "I do just 60 watts at 60 rpm (revolutions per minute) and gauge the distance based on my increase in heart rate," Bill maintained. Although Bill passed away in April 2010, at the very least, the sport gave him the opportunity to hope.

In addition to cycling's proven assets in cancer recovery, benefits for cancer prevention have also been documented. A recent Swedish paper published in the *British Journal of Cancer* reports that cycling as little as 30 minutes per day reduces the risk of cancer by 34 percent. This study evaluated more than 40,000 Scandinavian men, aged 45 to 79. The more time they spent cycling, the lower their risk of being diagnosed with cancer. Researchers compared responses from men with seven years of medical records with the group's 3,700 cancer cases to statistically qualify this correlation. In addition to reducing the incidence of cancer, cyclists who trained daily were 33 percent more likely to survive and recover from cancer. For each hour of moderate exercise, risk of cancer mortality dropped by 12 percent. Although increased activity leads to a longer life, medical professionals, who are traditionally conservative, also point out that the exact effects of exercise on cancer are still uncertain. Those of us who bike regularly have experienced the abundance of other health benefits, including increased cardiorespiratory health, reduced stress levels, and weight control.

Older masters cyclists are at even greater risk for bone damage than younger cyclists, according to a 2003 study by the International Osteoporosis and National Osteoporosis Foundations. Responses from a questionnaire on the history of leisure activity were used to correlate weight-bearing exercise and the bone-mineral densities (BMD) of three groups of men: older masters cyclists, at an average age of 51, who had trained for at least 10 years with little or no weight-bearing exercise; 16 younger cyclists, at an average age of 32, who had engaged in a minimum of weight-bearing exercise, and 24 nonathletes of a similar age and weight to the masters cyclists. DXA (dual-energy x-ray absorptiometry), which directs two x-ray beams with differing energy levels at the patients' bones, measured BMD of the spine and hip. The BMD of the bones can be determined by subtracting the soft-tissue absorption from the total value of the absorption of each beam. The results showed that the BMDs of the masters cyclists were significantly lower than those of the other two groups. "Although highly trained and physically fit," the report stated, "these athletes may be at high risk for developing osteoporosis with advancing age."

Weight-bearing exercise is not the only component necessary for healthy bones. Cyclists must eat sufficiently and sensibly to offset the calories they burn and to make sure they are supporting their bones with the proper nutrients. Hard-training female athletes who do not eat a good, nutritional diet can suffer from cessation of the menses, and bone loss. Poor nutrition can also interfere with the production of estrogen and testosterone, which help to slow the rate of bone loss in both sexes.

Increased Ability to Recover From Injury

Cycling is often used to rehabilitate knees after an injury or surgery. Therapeutic cycling is usually done on a stationary bicycle to avoid placing excessive loads on the joints. The continuous pedaling motion helps joints recover their former range of motion and may even improve it. Cycling therapy stimulates the production of synovial fluid, a viscous liquid that keeps the joints lubricated and nourished, preventing further damage. Cycling also stabilizes joints by strengthening the supporting musculature and can also address the stiffness and discomfort that accompany degenerative ailments like osteoarthritis.

Cycling offers an option for cross-training; for example, if runners recovering from injury need to avoid the impact that their sport inflicts on the joints, they can maintain their physical conditioning while allowing their injury to heal completely. Joan Benoit Samuelson, winner of the 1984 women's marathon in the Los Angeles Summer Olympics, spent the final weeks before the race training on a stationary bike to recover from knee surgery. After winning the PGA Masters tournament in 2008, Tiger Woods underwent knee surgery to repair the ACL in his left knee, and then began a rehabilitation program of stationary cycling, water exercise, and light strength training. He returned to tournament play in less than a year.

All workouts inflict at least a small degree of damage on the joints, muscles, and connective tissues; however, with sufficient recovery time, the affected tissues will not only heal but will also become stronger and less susceptible to future damage. Cycling allows athletes to take a break from sports that are more punishing physically without losing the level of fitness they have worked so hard to achieve.

LIFESTYLE CHALLENGES OF THE OLDER ATHLETE

As masters athletes age, their priorities change, and athletic pursuits take a back seat to more pressing responsibilities. Of course, this does not apply to older professionals or elite amateurs whose earnings depend on racing during the season and coaching during the off-season. The vast majority of masters, however, have significant demands on their time, such as families or full-time jobs unrelated to cycling. Many masters cyclists struggle to get enough time in the saddle while meeting their other obligations. The good news is that you can work full-time, fulfill your family responsibilities, and still have time to ride your bike if you manage your time creatively.

Finding the Time to Ride

Masters cyclists with families and careers confront more demands on their time than ever before. In most families with children, one or both parents work. They are also responsible for getting their kids to and from school, day care, and extracurricular activities. Meals must be prepared, homework must be supervised, and time must be set aside for activities involving the entire family. Finding time for cycling and other training requires a team approach from family members. Look at training as setting a positive example for the physical development and health of both kids and adults.

My friend and Olympic gold medalist Steve Hegg is a good example of how good parenting and cycling can work to benefit both parent and child, in this

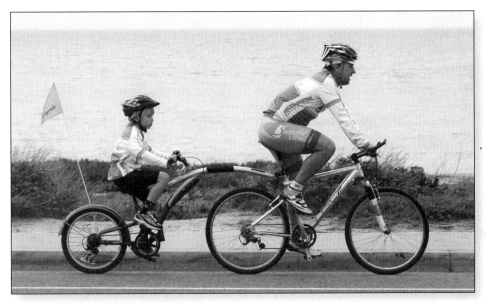

1984 Olympic gold medalist Steve Hegg and his son spend time together while cycling.

case, his son. Steve's competitive years are probably postponed or behind him, but his ability to maintain his cycling form while being a full-time dad to Jack is commendable. Steve added a child-carrier seat to his bicycle as soon as Jack was old enough to ride behind him. Jack is nearly 6 years old, and I have seen him cranking a pedal-extension device that Steve attached to his tandem. He is growing up with cycling and is developing a strong sense of discipline, which is a key factor in athletic performance at any age. Although not a father myself, I see riding a tandem with your youngster as an opportunity to bond and establish yourself as a positive role model.

Most masters cyclists work outside the home; many have families, and older masters cyclists, whose children may be grown, may have grandchildren to spoil and aging parents to care for. Whatever your circumstances, you may find yourself literally wedging your cycling workouts between the already jam-packed elements of work and family. To get your training in, you must adopt a good work ethic, a sense of discipline, and a measure of denial if you are going to compete with a high level of success. You may need to rise an hour earlier in the morning to get in a 15-minute core warm-up drill, followed by 30 minutes on your bike or trainer. I will explain the unique advantages of riding stationary rollers for this workout, but the real key to making the workout happen in the first place is to get sufficient sleep (record that favorite TV show and get to bed earlier). You can look forward to a heightened energy level in all facets of your life.

A sense of satisfaction will begin to build with daily and varied workouts. These energizing intervals are a great way to jump-start your metabolism early in the day. I personally find that they help me maintain my athleticism even if I cannot get in any other exercise that day. If you struggle with mornings, leave for work too early to train in the morning, or prefer your workouts later in the day, you will need to make similar adjustments in your daily routine. On days that I have commitments in the mornings, I find that a strong sense of discipline is necessary to fit in a workout later in the day, especially if the days are short and the sun sets early. An evening session on the trainer or a spin class seems to work for many masters cyclists. If you postpone your workout until too late in the evening, you may find that hard anaerobic or aerobic training makes it more difficult to sleep. Whenever you choose to work out, morning or evening, I guarantee you will feel good about yourself.

Integrating Cycling Into Your Lifestyle

Another way to get that aerobic workout is to commute by bicycle. Rob Macleod, author of *Rob's Bike Page* for *Cycling Utah* and member of the Mayor's Bicycle Advisory Committee in Salt Lake City, says, "Commuting is a sport." I like that definition. In a sense, turning commuting into a sport puts a new spin on the activity and the character of the participants. Rob is a daily, year-round commuter in Salt Lake City, Utah, a city not known for its mild winters. I have been a regular bicycle commuter most of my life and consider this one of the best ways

Link Lindquist

So you think you're too old to start cycling. Think again! Link Lindquist came to me for a bike fit at age 78 after he had been riding a bicycle for just about four years. He and his wife, Kathy, were already leading bike tours in Europe. Although Link was a very fit touring cyclist, I suggested that he try racing. He wasn't terribly enthusiastic about the idea at first but decided to race a year later and continued to do so over the next three years. He won the prestigious San Diego Omnium twice. After attending one of my skills courses, he won the triple crown of masters cycling by collecting gold in the road race, time trial, and criterium at the U.S. National Championships in Louisville, Kentucky. Link added to his list of victories in the National Senior Olympics in Palo Alto, California. He placed first in the 20K and 40K road

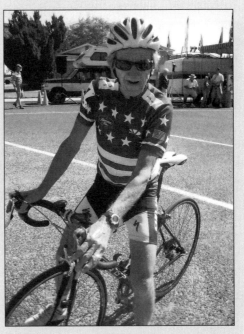

Link Lindquist, one of the world's fastest octogenarians.

races and second in the 5K and 10K time trials. To cap off the event, he finished in the top 10 in the 20K road race against much younger opponents.

As Link has done more training and acquired more racing experience, the way he trains has changed accordingly. "I've increased my use of interval training, and I'm riding with a faster group now. I've increased the plyometric training with box jumping and spend more time with the jump rope," he says. "I had to learn about mass-start racing, something that can be intimidating for a rookie. At the National Senior Games, there was a group start of more than 70 cyclists, and it helped me to become more comfortable with it."

Link's goals are a podium finish in the UCI Masters World Championships in Tirol, Austria. He would also like to win all the events he enters at the Huntsman World Games in St. George, Utah and to become the best age-category cyclist in the world. Outside of racing, Link appreciates what cycling has brought to his life. Link says that he has been able to maintain his weight, flexibility, agility, body fat, and aerobic capacity. He loves to jump rope and credits it with helping him to stay in shape and building his bone density.

"Cycling gives me the chance to ride my bike and take care of my body at the same time. It will also help me to achieve my long-term goal of running the Western States 100-Mile Endurance Run at age 100. The hardest thing about cycling is having to stay off the bike for two days a week!"

for serious cyclists to log miles. Commuting requires occasional sprint intervals and quick reflexes, thereby helping cyclists hone their bike-handling skills.

During my days as a college student, I learned the challenges and the sense of adventure associated with year-round commuting. I rode my bike daily to Southwest Missouri State in Springfield, up through the foothills of the Ozarks, sucking the smell of freshly cut grass through my nostrils on balmy spring days. My tires spun on wet leaves as I rode through a radiant bonfire of fall colors. I left my tire tracks in freshly fallen snow and picked my way through crusty ice on brutally cold mornings. I rode through the worst Missouri winter conditions, flaunting my bike's presence on the road and leaving my prized E-type Jaguar parked in the garage.

As gasoline prices have risen over the years, people have rediscovered bicycles as an economical way to get from point A to point B. Unfortunately, most of the people who are fed up with the price of fuel and choose to boycott the driving experience soon relent and return to their cars when the prices at the pump begin to drop. Many cyclists ride for the joy of the physical exertion that riding a bicycle offers and for its value as an ecological activity. Most bike commuters enjoy the ability to unwind guilt-free after a hectic workday and to get a workout in the process. A survey of 2,400 cyclists who commute on a regular basis revealed the following commonalities:

- 95 percent ride for health and fitness.
- 82 percent want to preserve the environment.
- 52 percent like to bike to avoid traffic congestion.
- 46 percent want to save money on fuel.
- 34 percent want to avoid the cost and inconvenience of parking.

The average bicycle commuter in North America is male, 39 years of age, and a professional. Senior citizens in the United States make only 9 percent of their trips by cycling or walking, but in Germany and the Netherlands, seniors make more than half of their excursions by cycling or walking.

Commuting in cold conditions requires mental toughness to endure windchill, snow, ice, and varying road conditions, all of which will make you appreciate the spring and summer commutes that much more. When temperatures drop to near or below freezing, ice may be present; adjust your speed accordingly. Motorists will have more difficulty seeing out of frosted windows, especially when just starting their cars or driving in bright sunlight. With high snow banks, visibility becomes even more of an issue, so it would be wise to adopt a defensive attitude. During short winter days, maximize your visibility by wearing bright clothing and a good helmet. If you ride at night, wear reflective clothing and use a high-intensity lighting system to aid your visibility in the dark. Most nighttime accidents occur because cyclists are invisible to motorists, so if you commute by the light of the moon, do not trust that you will be seen.

If you intend to ride in adverse conditions, a certain amount of defensive training may save you from crashing in an actual emergency situation. Practice negotiating icy or slick roads by finding an empty parking lot or quiet street on which to experiment with maneuvers that will give you a better idea of what your limits are. If commuting on rough roads or in extreme winter conditions is part of your adventure, install tires with thick, deep treads or knobbies. If you are a purist, you may want to have a set of wheels with metal studded tires mounted up and ready to go.

If you are commuting in a cold climate, you must wear a windproof outer layer, especially if you have any long descents. Build your clothing in thin layers, with a layer of polypropylene next to your skin to wick away sweat. Climbing a grade may leave you wet, but wicking materials will help you avoid hypothermia (a drop in body core temperature to 95 degrees Fahrenheit or less) in cold temperatures. Years ago, we used breathable wool underneath our outerwear, but the lightweight miracle fibers available today are superior in all regards. There is nothing worse than a cold, clammy layer of cotton next to your skin. Be prepared to shed or add layers as the temperatures and conditions shift. Always carry or have dry clothing available to change into after arriving at your destination.

Unless you are an equipment junkie, you will not need anything exotic for commuting. Many commuters have a bike they modify specifically for that purpose, and they can outfit it with fenders, lights, and panniers. I sometimes commute on a single-speed bicycle, which puts me right out in the street with the current crop of single-speed cultists. My favorite rides are typically on my oldest collector bikes from the 1950s and '60s. Some of the bikes from this era are equipped with eyelets for fenders and pannier bags. Older bikes for commuting are very easy to find online or in your local newspaper. Prices start at $20 USD and go up from there. The most remarkable finds seem to come from garage sales, which is how I acquired most of the steel bikes in my collection. Steel bikes work fine in San Diego but may not be the best choice in winter, especially if the streets are salted, since mild steel will rust.

Macleod recommends scaling up slowly in poor conditions. For beginning commuters, the first challenge is to be comfortable on your bike in traffic, a subject that will be covered in depth later. John Coble, a friend and fellow commuter, suggests doing some research and experimentation with your route to find the passages that are the safest, most expeditious, and more scenic. John, who commutes into Washington D.C., shuns the main traffic routes and takes a bike path into the capitol.

Commuting or training rides in traffic can be a lot safer if some general rules are observed. First of all, be sure to behave in a predictable manner, making no sudden or abrupt moves. Behave as though you are a motorist and observe all traffic laws. If you are in an intersection and will be proceeding straight through it, don't block motorists who are waiting to make a right turn. Pull into the left turn lane to make a left turn; do not turn across multiple lanes of traffic. Ride in the same direction as the traffic and not against it like a pedestrian. Always signal your intentions, but never assume that motorists see you, and proceed with caution. For more information, refer to Web sites like http://www.bikexprt .com and http://www.bikeleague.org (League of American Bicyclists).

Commuting by Bike: Did You Know?

- Commuting by bicycle can result in 13 lbs (6 kg) of weight loss for the average person after one year.
- The risk for heart disease can be decreased by 50 percent by riding a bicycle three hours per week.
- A cyclist who weighs 140 lbs (63 kg) and pedals 14 miles (23 km) in an hour can burn 508 calories.
- If bicycle trips rose from 1.0 percent to 1.5 percent of all trips, 462,000,000 gallons (1,748.860244 L) of gas could be saved in the United States each year.
- People who commute by car sit in traffic for an average of 50 hours each year.
- Five billion gallons of fuel were burned by people sitting in rush-hour traffic in 2003.
- In 1964, 50 percent of children rode their bikes to school and obesity was at 12 percent.
- In 2004, only 3 percent of children biked to school, and obesity was 45 percent.
- Sixty percent of car pollution occurs during the first few minutes after a car is started.
- Twenty-five percent of all trips are 1 mile (1.6 km) or less from home, 40 percent are 2 miles (3 km) or less, and 50 percent of commuters live within 5 miles (8 km) of work.

Source: www.1world2wheels.org. One world two wheels is a trademark of Trek Bicycle Corporation.

Finally, no pitch for commuting would be complete without highlighting one of the best reasons for cycling to work: improving the environment. Cycling decreases traffic congestion and air pollution while reducing the need for parking. Motorists who are hostile to cyclists should appreciate the advantages that they enjoy with fewer cars on the road. Cyclists would be wise to act as ambassadors on the road. Always behave in a courteous manner when commuting by bike and follow the rules of the road. The motorist you antagonize today may take it out on another cyclist tomorrow. Whether I'm running or cycling, I make it a point to wave to a motorist who has patiently waited for me before proceeding.

Seeking Out Friendly Options for Masters

If the idea of commuting by bike leaves you cold (figuratively or literally), or you want additional opportunities to increase your level of fitness and improve your riding skills while having fun, join a bike club. Most group cycling starts at the club level. During group rides, you learn to ride in close proximity to others, draft, ride in a pace line, and develop your bike-handling skills. Your fitness level, strength-to-weight ratio, and availability will determine the group you ride with. Most clubs have groups of varying abilities, and you may find that you progressively advance from one to the next as your skill level and endurance improves. There is great camaraderie among club members, and the stronger riders inspire the less-skilled riders to challenge themselves.

Historically, cycling in the United States has been a club sport. Clubs exist throughout the country, and most cater to masters racers. Some, like San Diego Cyclo-Vets and Carolina Masters Cycling, feature special events especially for masters in age categories. As I previously mentioned, bicycle racing in the United States is essentially a masters sport with categories starting at age 30. Many top masters racers also race in the elite categories. The ability of top masters racers to ride with top professional riders is perhaps the most unique feature of U.S. cycling. In Europe, the ranking system is far more restricted, and the categories of elite and masters are not as interchangeable. Masters cyclists have an array of events, including road racing; subcategories of criteriums, or circuit racing; and time trials. Mountain-bike events include subcategories of cross-country, downhill, and time trials.

However, frustrations do exist among masters in the older categories. Kenton, my friend and training client, is 70 and enters bike races to improve his time-trial speed. He is a top age-group triathlete on the U.S. national team. Kenton and I both agree that too few opportunities exist for older masters to compete. As one ages, the traditional five-year increments become more and more critical. Although many race promoters offer a 40-plus and sometimes a 50-plus category, few events cater to riders in their 60s and beyond, and these categories are growing rapidly. "Running, swimming, and triathlons have spoiled masters into feeling we should be pampered with our own exclusive five-year brackets," Kenton says wistfully. He became serious about cycling when he was trying to rebuild his strength and endurance after an automobile accident some years ago. Masters cycling has become an increasingly difficult sport for scoring wins, as Kenton has discovered. "As a licensed rider, I have very rarely placed in a bike race, but I am still trying. There are other masters in their 70s who won't enter anything since they can't find their age bracket on the registration form."

You can choose from many racing genres, such as time trials, road and track racing, mountain biking, and cyclo-cross. If racing doesn't appeal to you, plenty of cycling activities exist with varying degrees of difficulty to accommodate your preferences and skill level, including centuries and multiple-day tours. You can also change your scenery in a pedaled watercraft.

Time Trials

If you are thinking about entering a bicycle race for the first time, start out with a time trial. Time trials are easy to enter, and the choice of equipment is completely up to you. Time-trial coverage on television shows cyclists with very specialized equipment that is literally shaped by the wind. This is because the faster you ride, the larger the factor wind resistance becomes. For example, when you are cruising along at 10 miles per hour on a flat road, it doesn't take a lot of effort to maintain speed; however, if you are riding that same road at 20 mph, around 80 percent of your effort is used to combat wind resistance. Equipment that is specifically designed to reduce this effect, such as the lightweight bikes with aerodynamic frames, skin suits, aero wheels, and aero helmets that you see the pros wear are available for purchase, but don't feel you have to spend a lot of money to explore this disciplined type of racing. If you can afford a little equipment, start with clip-on aero bars and an aerodynamic helmet, which will give you the most bang for your buck. The bars will allow you to tuck into an aerodynamic position, which will significantly reduce the effort you have to expend to maintain speed. According to *Peak Performance*, a British website that is devoted to competitive sports, a cyclist who is sitting up in the saddle will need to produce 340 watts of power to maintain a speed of 22 mph. However, if he or she assumes a tucked position on the bike, the power output needed to maintain speed drops to 170 watts. For this reason, aerobars are at the top of the equipment list for time trialists.

Typically, time trials take place on courses that are flat or slightly rolling. Riders are staged in intervals that range from 30 seconds to one minute. Many events held across the country and around the globe cater to masters racers. Refer to websites, such as www.USAcycling.org, ambikerace.com, and others, to locate the events in or near your area.

If you want to take your pace-line skills to another level in a competitive environment, try the team time trial (TTT). In U.S. competition, four riders usually work together to quickly pace their way through a 40K course. State TTT championships for various age categories are becoming increasingly popular.

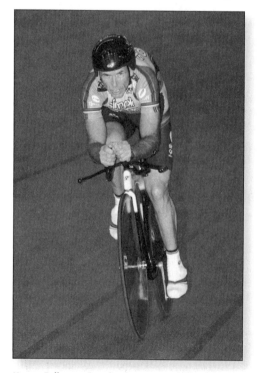

Kenny Fuller setting the masters world hour record at the AEG Home Depot velodrome in Carson, California.

Road and Track Racing

Although time trials should be a part of your regular training regimen, the next rung on the ladder is the road race. Road racing is the essence of cycling and features venues with a huge variety of terrain and courses. This type of race allows you to test your riding skills and fitness gains while avoiding dangerous, close-contact races, such as criteriums. You will discover your strengths and weaknesses on certain courses and will learn to adjust your training to compensate. Road racing will test your limits and will satisfy your competitive desires.

Track racing is another venue to consider, and many major cities have velodromes. The main Olympic categories include pursuit, match sprinting, and team racing. At many velodromes worldwide, the focus has switched from racing to recreational training. Riding a fixed-gear bike on a banked track is an incredibly exciting experience. With basic instruction, this type of training is ideal for road riders. Great road sprinters like Mark Cavendish refined their technique for stage-winning sprints by riding on the track. My best sprints and several of my victories at masters national championships can be attributed to my group workouts at the San Diego velodrome.

Multiple-Day Tours

Multiple-day tours are another way to increase your endurance and cycling skills while having fun. You can choose tours for mountain biking or road cycling. These tours usually involve traveling to a starting location, riding a predetermined distance each day, camping or staying in arranged accommodations, and returning to the starting point with tour guides. Meals are usually included in the price. Tours can last from two days to a week, or longer, and some linger for several days in a particular location to allow time for sightseeing. The fees for one Italian bike tour include travel to the starting point, full van support, four-star accommodations, wine tasting, and a commemorative jersey.

Although they are billed as tours, many rides can be fairly competitive, as my friend and fellow masters rider, Judy, found during a recent tour in the Pyrenees with her boyfriend, Jim. "We had a GPS, so we were self sufficient and really enjoyed the scenery. In the mountains, the young testosterone-driven guys just rode away from us and beat each other up. They were all former racers. You never really know who is going to sign up for these smaller rides." Therefore, riding with a smaller tour group may prove to be either a wonderful training experience or an exercise in frustration, depending on your level of ability. It may be prudent to train for the specific requirements of the ride and ask the organizers about the number, riding experience, and ages of participants before signing on. Ask about GPS mapping and custom

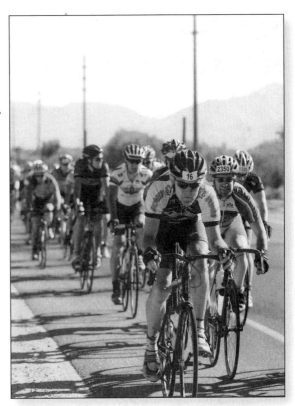

John Howard leading the pack in El Tour de Tucson, 2009.

tours and, for safety's sake, about the number of support vehicles and support personnel that will be present, as well as their qualifications. On the larger multiday tours, many levels of ability are usually represented, and you are less likely to be left behind.

Century Rides

Whether you race or not, it helps to set a goal as your mileage base develops. Since the early days of the sport in the late 1800s, when the League of American Wheelmen was actively lobbying state and national governments to build hard surface roads, the century ride has become a rite of passage for cyclists of all age categories. Century rides are 100 miles (161 km) in length. Metric centuries of 100 kilometers (about 62 miles) also exist. Set your sights on one of the many available events as you train. I have found that ultradistance enthusiasts are usually easygoing cyclists who have a lot of fun. Ultradistance rides, based on skill level and experience, often do not require qualification.

Pedaled Watercraft

Although cycling in the traditional sense involves pedaling to cover ground, pedaling propulsion is not limited to bicycles. Some of the most enjoyable cycling experiences can take place without a helmet or wheels. Pedaled watercrafts have been around for some time, but don't mistake the newer, sleek crafts for the cumbersome paddleboats you may have ridden at resorts. A new generation of hydrodynamic pedal crafts is available that includes the fastest human-powered watercrafts on the planet. The craft with the latest technology has a powerful propeller that is driven by rotational pedaling and has a rudder for steering. It also operates in forward and reverse. Technique, coordination,

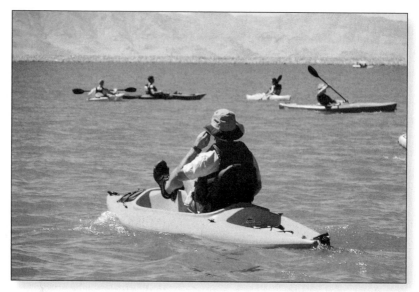

The Wavewalker pedal-driven boat at Lake Travis in Austin, Texas.

and training are not prerequisites for operating these crafts. The experience of exploring fresh or salt waterways in one of these fine boats is invigorating, refreshing, and physically challenging. You don't need to worry about cars, and the boats are lightweight and easy to launch. If you're interested in kayak fishing, pedal-powered boats offer hands-free propulsion. Rod racks, fish-finders, drink holders, ample cargo storage, and deck space are generally abundant on most of the new crafts. The better units feature out-of-water storage and retractable skids for navigating shallow water.

Mountain Biking

Another fun form of cycling is mountain biking. Just as you worked to build an endurance base and bike-handling skills for road cycling, you would be wise to acquire some basic skills before venturing onto more-advanced technical trails. You might find joining a mountain-biking club helpful, but you can also network online or tap the resources at your local bike shop. You can acquire descending, climbing, and cornering skills from progressive practice, but instruction accelerates the process. It is my belief that technical instruction is as important for mountain biking as it is for any other sport. Once you can descend a fire trail or a tricky single track at a comfortable speed, you can explore so much more of the natural world. The off-road environment is very enjoyable, filled with beautiful scenery and devoid of noisy traffic.

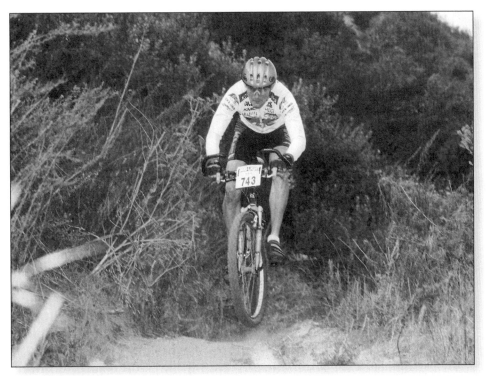

John Howard getting air time while mountain biking.

BMX

BMX is another form of off-road cycling. The precise origin is uncertain; however, Bruce Brown's classic 1971 motorcycle film, *On Any Sunday*, is generally credited with inspiring the BMX movement. The sport's roots also extend worldwide, not just to Canada and Australia. BMX had its beginnings as a children's sport, but now many middle-aged cyclists ride the twisting little tracks, catching air. The sport played on the world stage at the 2008 Summer Olympic Games in Beijing and at the X-Games. Introduce your kids to BMX. Many of the top road and off-road racers have BMX pedigrees. If you spend even a small percentage of your cycling time off-road, you are adding another dimension to this sport for life.

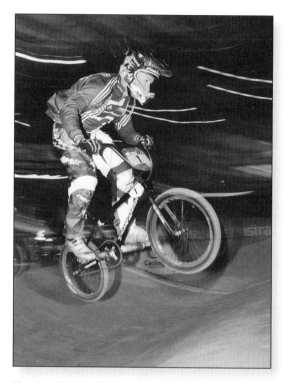

Five-time UCI World Champion Dale Holmes competing in BMX at the Beijing Olympics in 2008.

TECHNOLOGICAL ADVANCES IN CYCLING

One of the many appealing aspects of the bicycle is its simple mechanical efficiency and its place in the evolution of the motorcycle, the automobile, and the airplane. Henry Ford, founder of the first practical mass-produced automobile, was a bicycle mechanic who borrowed bicycle parts and designs for his model A Ford. The Wright brothers were also bicycle-shop mechanics who solved complex aeronautical problems with simple bicycle components. This type of thinking continued into World War II, when the landing-gear return assembly on a period fighter plane consisted of a hand-operated bike chain and a sprocket. Like a lot of American assembly facilities, the Schwinn bicycle factory in Chicago turned out airplane parts for the war effort. Schwinn bikes from that era reveal a wonderful array of machines with the look and feel of motorcycles and airplanes. Today, these toy machines are some of the most sought-after collectibles in the vintage bicycle market. This heritage is seen in the lightweight racing and touring bikes of today.

Aero Bars

The move to modernize cycling by making bikes aerodynamic is historically rooted in the 1890s, when cyclist and machinist, Marshall "Major" Taylor, created an innovative sliding outrigger stem that enabled the black star to slide into a tucked racing position, giving him an edge over his competition. In the 1930s, Oscar Egg, a Swiss track cyclist, built a radical aerodynamic bicycle fairing and a recumbent pilot that enabled him to set bicycle speed records, including the world hour record. In 1984, Francesco Moser used an innovative, low-front disc wheel on his bike that allowed him to easily break Eddy Merckx's historic 1972 world hour record with a speed of 31.78 mph (51 kph). Although the practice was not yet illegal in international competition when he did it, blood-doping later tainted his effort. With the exception of the low-slung, bullet-shaped racing machines designed by members of the International Human-Powered Vehicle Association, which were not allowed in competitions, the aero movement didn't gain much ground until the 1980s.

Aerodynamic handlebars were first conceived by Jim Elliott, Race Across America (RAAM) rider, and Richard Bryne of Speedplay Pedals. In 1986, Pete Penseyres developed a prototype aero-bar system to win his third RAAM. The bars were redesigned by Chester Kyle, a mechanical-engineering professor at California State University in Long Beach. Scott Gordon, engineer of Aero Sports, constructed them from balsa wood and aluminum. Pete also used a very early carbon-fiber, rear-disc wheel designed by Kyle and Gordon in the 1986 RAAM where he set a speed record that still stands at 15.4 mph (25 kph). The 3,107-mile (5,000 km) race took him eight days and nine hours to complete.

A variety of production aero handlebars soon appeared, first on the bikes ridden by innovation-seeking triathletes, then on Greg LeMond's time-trial bike in 1989 at the Tour de France. Greg won the final time-trial stage and the Tour by a mere eight seconds over French favorite Laurent Fignon. This margin was certainly due to the aero bars, disc wheel, and pointed aero helmet, which he wore at a time when most Tour riders raced bareheaded. Today, aero bars and aero wheels are common on time-trial bikes. Aerodynamic frames, spoke systems, skin suits, booties, and drinking systems have also evolved in low-speed wind tunnels, a practical place for testing aero equipment for pro teams and a few of the best-funded masters racers. Nothing is more satisfying than riding a beautifully crafted machine that enables you to travel quietly across the landscape at 15 to 25 miles per hour (24-40 kph) or more. Feeling the wind in your face and the blood pulsing through your body is an exhilarating sensation.

Training Tools

Advances in technology do not stop with the bicycle. Masters athletes who are serious about their training can use heart-rate monitoring devices, power meters, and GPS technologies to aid them in gauging their progress. According to Hunter Allen and Andrew Coggan, authors of *Training and Racing with a Power Meter*, the indoor power meter, or ergometer, has been around since the late 1800s. This fact surprised me. Power meters and heart-rate monitors (HRMs) can be effectively used to improve your understanding of the aerobic and anaerobic variables that enable you to train more effectively. Power meters can be used to better understand functional threshold power and how it is affected by heart rate, blood-lactate levels, and wattage. Most power meters use strain gauges to measure torque and angular velocity, which are then used to calculate power. This type of power meter has been available since the late 1980s and is mounted on the bottom bracket, crankset, or rear hub. Power meters that are more modern measure certain Newtonian forces, including wind and rolling resistance, inertia, and gravity. In conjunction with velocity, they calculate the power output of the rider in watts. These meters are mounted on the bike's handlebars. It should be mentioned that power meters are expensive, costing anywhere from almost $700 to $2,300 USD. HRMs are a more affordable alternative but can't provide information on power output. Using a sensor that is held in place with a strap on the chest, the heart rate of the wearer is displayed on a wrist-mounted unit. The basic models record your maximum heart rate, average heart rate and allow you to program the unit to beep when you fall below your target heart rate. Many also function as watches and will display the calories burned during a workout. Although our bodies are amazingly efficient, their power potential is about the same as a row of four 75-watt incandescent light bulbs. Consider using multiple methodologies for fine-tuning your technique for maximum performance.

Technology can also be used to make workouts more fun and to provide needed information. Cyclometers have been around for decades. Using a sensor that is attached to the frame, they register the speed, distance, and elevation changes during your ride and store cumulative gains in mileage and altitude. Some offer benefits similar to the GPS and have cadence sensors, HRMs, and USB interfaces. GPS systems, some of which come with heart-rate monitors, allow you to download your ride onto your desktop or laptop computer and keep an ongoing log of your workouts. This powerful tool records your actual route and elevation changes so that you can look at a satellite or street map of your ride and a profile of the topography. Mapping technology is a great way to share your rides with others. For a thrill, import a ride into the Internet program Google Earth and view the route, first from outer space and zooming in up close.

Advantages of the cyclometer include longer battery life and more accurate measurements of distance and speed. Because they don't rely on maintaining satellite contact among tall buildings or in dense stands of trees, cyclometers are generally less expensive. You also don't have to wait the 30 seconds it usually takes to establish satellite contact when using them. Other benefits of some GPS models include freedom from attached sensors, display of street maps and directions, and other multisport applications.

Older masters cyclists truly appreciate the technological developments the sport has seen since they can recall the days when gear levers were on the down tube and shift-index systems didn't exist. They remember the awkwardness of toe clips and having to estimate the mileage they covered and the elevation gained during a training ride. The number of available gears and the protection offered by helmets have increased dramatically. Those who compete can appreciate the improved aerodynamics and the lighter bycycle frames available today. They also have fun with the plethora of gadgets that enhance the training experience.

Although masters cyclists confront challenges associated with their lifestyles and aging, most of the issues can be resolved or reduced to tolerable levels so that cycling remains a beneficial and enjoyable sport throughout their lives.

Essential Bike Setup

A bicycle is a compound machine, a system of levers and pulleys with key components that must be adjusted to increase power and comfort for the rider. There is a clear distinction between sizing and fitting. Sizing is the process of finding the right frame size, and fitting is the process of maximizing your comfort and power by fine-tuning the adjustable components of the bike. When it comes to finding the right frame size, I recommend seeking the advice of your local bike dealer. Please keep in mind that while a good bike fit adjusts the bike to the rider, a great fit should do more. The biomechanical deficiencies of the rider must also be addressed. You may be acutely aware when things are not right with your bike setup, but many cyclists do not realize they have adjustment flaws until they begin to feel pain in their knees, hips, and backs.

In their book *Bike for Life*, Roy Wallack and Bill Katovsky maintain that good pain leads to high performance when the cyclist and the bike are indistinguishable from one another and are working in harmony. This pain is associated with the muscle-strengthening process, the cost that is exacted for performance gains. Pain in the knees, back, hips, crotch, wrist, or hands is classified as bad. This pain is debilitating, discouraging, and interferes with the quality of your cycling. When we experience acute discomfort, we tend to avoid the activity that causes it. You can avoid most of these painful issues if your bike is the right size and is adjusted to accommodate you. However, both stationary and mobile bicycles can injure their occupants or aggravate existing injuries if they are not properly fitted.

BASICS OF FITTING

A successful bike setup strikes a balance of power, comfort, and sustained endurance. If you are a road racer, a time trialist, racing in criteriums, or a recreational enthusiast, there are subtle variations in the way the bike is adjusted, but they are essentially similar to one another. The amount of cycling experience the rider has may influence the aggressiveness of his or her position on the bike. Also, everyone rides in traffic at some point, and a good setup will allow you to maneuver through it safely and confidently. Your torso should rest on the saddle, supported lightly by the arms and hands, and your weight should be neutrally balanced (see figure 3.1). You should not feel impingement in your hips, spine, neck, shoulders, arms, or hands. The muscles of the quadriceps in the upper leg and the hip flexors in the groin share the load in stabilizing the legs, and both legs should equally share the motions of lifting and pushing while maintaining a straight plane.

In the best position, your feet should rest flat (no supination or pronation) on the pedals parallel to one another. This is a departure from the traditional ideology of correct positioning. At one time, it was maintained that the shoe/pedal interface should be allowed to track in a "natural" pattern. This concept was supported by the subsequent development and promotion of cleats and pedals that allowed the feet to float on the pedals. It was a widely publicized belief that a splayed foot, hence a splayed knee, is a natural physical feature; however, this is usually not true. This anomaly is most often due

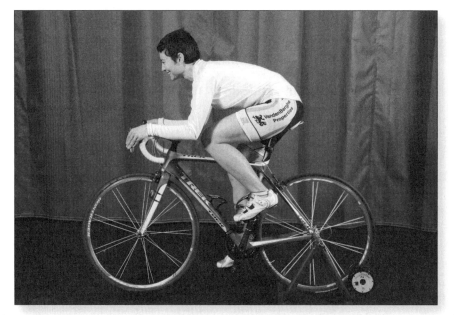

Figure 3.1 Profile of rider in correct tucked position: The pelvis is tilted down slightly, the spine is neutral, the elbows are bent, and the hands are draped over the brake lever hoods.

to tight iliotibial bands and/or tight external hip rotators, both of which can be easily corrected. The most efficient means of transferring power from the legs through the pedals by the feet is perpendicular to the cranks. Cyclists who race and those who ride recreationally are abandoning the floating pedals because they rob them of power, and their bodies work more efficiently with a disciplined pedal stroke.

A neutral spine and a slight forward tilt of the pelvic girdle allow the elbows to bend naturally. In this position, you can engage the core muscles and provide a stable platform for the primary muscles: the quadriceps, hamstrings, and glutes. This produces more power while reducing heart rate and oxygen demand, thus delaying the onset of fatigue. In addition to lowering the body profile and minimizing wind drag, this body position absorbs shock better because the torso is slightly lower and the elbows are bent. The shoulders will relax, and breathing will be rhythmic and less labored.

An efficient body position will not overuse any one muscle group. Many masters cyclists complain of discomfort in the lower back, especially after long rides. This may indicate that they are not engaging all of their core muscles equally along with the psoas and the gluteus medius. This results in an overextension of the lower back. See figure 3.2 for an example of a correctly balanced body position. This chapter discusses the saddle in more depth in following sections, but it is worth noting here that saddle position is critical for a good fit. At the correct saddle height, joint angles open up and the primary muscles fire more efficiently. A good fitter adjusts the tilt of the saddle and the fore and aft

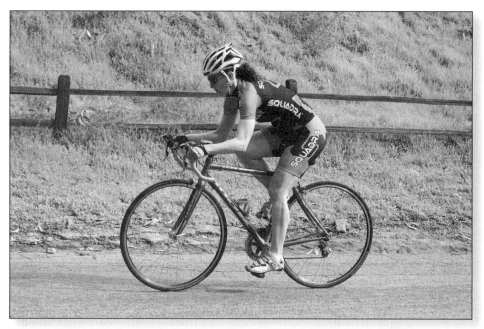

Figure 3.2 A balanced performance position.

(forward and backward) position to allow the cyclist to take better advantage of the biggest and most powerful muscle group in the body, the glutes. Strong gluteal muscles promote more efficient climbing with a smooth, powerful cadence, either out of the saddle or from a seated position for solo or group riding.

A road cyclist has five points of contact with the bike: the two pedals, the saddle, and the two handlebars. Aerodynamic time-trial cyclists and triathletes have additional contact points with the forearms. These points must be aligned to avoid fatigue and overuse of individual muscle groups. Various body dimensions vector power differently, and each cyclist is different. So it is impossible to rely on a system that defines absolute angles or percentages. The fundamental problem with conventional bike-store fittings is that they tend to ignore the anatomical function of individual bodies. Many mechanical adjustments fail to consider the biomechanical idiosyncrasies that occur with different physiques.

Dr. Ernie Ferrel is a sports chiropractor with more than 30 years of experience working with Olympic athletes, professional cyclists, amateurs, and masters cyclists. He and I have used a combination of body assessments and soft-tissue manipulation in our unique fitting system. We have found that hip and knee pain from overuse are the most common complaints among masters cyclists. Sixty-five percent of all riders report knee and hip pain during or after rides longer than 50 miles (80 km).

In physically active athletes, both anterior (front) and posterior (rear) ligaments provide maximum stability in extension and minimal stability in flexion. Extension is the act of increasing the angle between the bones of a limb at the joint; flexion is the decrease of that angle. When pedaling, both extension and flexion are occurring rapidly and simultaneously in the legs. An imbalance of the force applied to the pedals by each leg during the pedal stroke can cause disproportionate pressure to be applied to the hip joints and knees, resulting in microscopic tears to the tissue. This microtrauma can also be due to a sudden increase in the duration or intensity of cycling, especially in larger gears. Highly repetitive motion can lead to muscular imbalances and tightness of the capsules that protect synovial joints. Synovial joints, like knees, contain a fluid that lubricates and nourishes them, keeping them functioning smoothly. When the capsules are tight, the joint experiences excessive wear to the moving parts and becomes inflamed.

Another issue that is often overlooked is the existence of discrepancies in leg length. Differences in leg length can be congenital but are more commonly acquired through atrophy of soft tissue. Both conditions affect the outcome of a bike fit and must be addressed, the former with an orthotic or shimming and the latter with soft-tissue manipulation and regular stretching. Changes that result from scarring due to injuries or surgery can also affect a good fit. Medical professionals can identify and isolate problems by pinpointing the location of the pain. In cycling, the hip area is the most common starting point. Assuming the preceding issues have been or will be addressed by the professional fitting you, let's discuss the fitting process.

FITTING A BIKE

Masters cyclists who are looking for a correct fit should choose their fitter with care. Those with fewer than 10 years of experience or a thousand fits under their belt often lack the knowledge needed to understand the biomechanics involved with the vast array of body types, let alone the different types of bikes and their applications. Fitting is far more of a physical process than a mechanical one. The biomechanical issues that affect power, comfort, and efficiency are greatly influenced by the cyclist's age. Although the fitting process relies on the act of turning bolts, it must be based primarily on the elements of functional anatomy. As a serious masters cyclist, you should be able to tweak your own setup for maximum power, comfort, and safety. I will walk you through the process. First, you will need to gather the following items and someone to help you conduct your fit:

- Digital camera, computer, and printer
- Bike trainer
- Protractor and ruler
- Digital level
- Allen wrench
- Plumb line
- Electrician's tape or colored markers to mark changes
- Standard tape measure

Once you have gathered everything on the list, attach your bike to the trainer and make sure both the floor and the bike are level. Use the appropriate spacer for a 700 or 650 wheel. I will now guide you systematically through the setup process.

Assess Your Hamstring Flexibility

Hamstring flexibility indicates how much power you will have to generate wattage. Remove your shoes, stand with your knees and feet together, and plant your buttocks against the wall. Without bending your knees or back, reach for the floor. If you can comfortably place your palms flat on the floor, set the saddle to a position between 30 and 35 degrees, using the procedure described in the section on adjusting saddle height. If you have difficulty reaching the floor but can touch your feet, a position between 35 and 40 degrees will serve you well. If you cannot reach below your ankles, you will be limited to a position between 40 and 45 degrees until your active range of motion increases.

You should also note the importance of ankle flexibility. Train your pedal stroke by pointing your toe down at the bottom of the stroke. If you have ridden your bike in cruiser mode, using a low saddle height and leading with a heel stroke while pedaling for some time, you may need to stretch and practice the correct pedaling motion for several months before raising the saddle to a height that is more efficient. A flexible body delivers more power, and a few extra millimeters of height will help open up the hamstrings.

Mount Your Bike

Get on your bike and warm up for 10 minutes on the trainer, gradually increasing your rpm (revolutions per minute) for about five minutes. Using a digital camera, have a friend shoot a profile shot of you at the 6 o'clock and 3 o'clock positions of the pedal stroke (see figures 3.3a and 3.3b). The camera should be held on a flat plane, such as a tripod, or on any level surface. Print the photos.

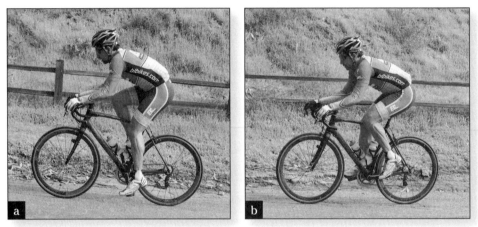

Figure 3.3   Cyclist's leg in (a) the 6 o'clock position and (b) the 3 o'clock position.

Adjust the Saddle Height

After taking the 6 o'clock photo, use a straight edge and protractor to draw and measure the angles intersecting the points of the various joints (see figure 3.4). The line along the inside centerline of the protractor should intersect the knee. Follow the white line of the upper leg to find the initial leg angle. Assess your flexibility and range and make the appropriate changes to your saddle (note that 10 degrees is approximately 2.5 centimeters).

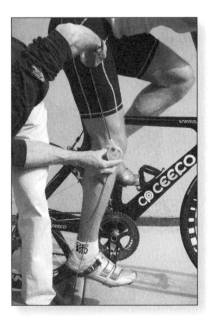

Figure 3.4   Measuring the fully extended leg in the 6 o'clock position.

Set the saddle and shoot another photo, rechecking as needed until you can feel your gluteal muscles firing as you ramp up your pedal stroke. If you are pedaling correctly, you should have a downward toe angle of approximately 15 to 20 degrees at the bottom of the stroke. You will engage the lower-leg muscles better during the recovery portion of your stroke, delivering power more consistently. The corresponding leg angle will generate the most power from your big muscles and will put the least amount of stress on your knees.

Fitting Variations for Different Bikes

The fitting method depends on the bike and how it will be ridden. For example, a road bike will be adjusted to a more aggressive position if the cyclist will be competing, especially for time trials that rely on aerodynamics. The bike can have a more aggressive adjustment for shorter time trials, such as the 40K bike split in an Olympic distance triathlon or the prologue in a stage race. The position for longer distances, such as half- or full-ironman bike splits, will be a little more relaxed for comfort. Since other individual issues may need to be accommodated, there are no hard and fast rules.

Mountain Bikes

Fitting mountain bikes is an exercise in transition. Although they employ many of the same power principles that apply to road bikes, such as saddle height, fore and aft position, and tilt positions, fitters must also consider the technical nature of trails. For example, a long, precipitous, rutted, or technically difficult trail requires that the saddle be positioned low and back for steep descents. Some mountain bikes come equipped with quick-release seat posts; if not, you can install one on your bike. Some are spring loaded, allowing you to make adjustments on the fly. At the very least, carry the correct size of Allen wrench when cycling so you can raise or lower your saddle as needed.

Hybrids and Commuter Bikes

Utilitarian bikes are not usually set up with performance in mind. Riders who commute may position their saddles lower for more comfort in traffic, which requires numerous mounts and dismounts. A commuter bike that is loaded with extra weight, such as fenders, panniers, or backpacks, will place additional stress on the rider's knees, which will already experience an increased burden from the lower saddle position. If your commute is longer than 10 miles (16 km) and you carry a load on your bike, you may want to experiment with saddle positions to find one that offers maximal comfort for the task.

Recumbents

The setup for recumbent riders most likely follows the same power principles as those for road cyclists. A prone seating position is the most comfortable and potentially powerful layout of any design. All of the human-powered speed records have been set with recumbent bikes.

Set the Fore and Aft Saddle Position

Drop a plumb line from the joint midline of the knee (see figure 3.5). Unless your lower leg (tibia) is disproportionately longer than your upper leg (femur), or the frame angles of the bike are exceptionally steep, the plumb line should fall across or near the ball of the foot and the pedal axle. For optimal time trialing with aero bars, adjust the saddle slightly forward so that your elbows and back are as flat as possible. In this position, the pivot point of the knee generally places the plumb line slightly ahead of the ball of the foot. The plumb angle is affected by the geometry of the frame and the length of the tibia (large bone in the lower leg) and the femur (upper-leg bone). A time-trial frame with an angle between 78 and 80 degrees brings the rider forward, throwing the plumb line in front of the ball of the foot. A longer tibia will have the same effect.

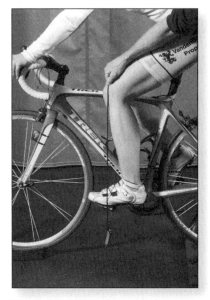

Figure 3.5 Leg in the 3 o'clock position with plumb line dropped.

Adjust the Seat Position (Nose Tilt)

Most cyclists notice the tilt of the saddle's nose before they feel changes in saddle height. A slight downward tilt to the saddle sets up a series of important biokinetic patterns for maximal power and comfort. The perfect tilt varies, depending on your flexibility, comfort zone, and choice of saddle. I recommend approximately 2 to 3 degrees of downward tilt. Adjust the nose using a digital level and an Allen wrench. The position of the saddle should feel completely neutral without excessive weight on the handlebars.

If, after riding for several minutes, you find yourself correcting the angle by sliding back, the nose is positioned too low. Fine-tuning your adjustments is easier when your bike has a microadjustable seat post, rather than the older cradle and spline type, so an upgrade may be necessary to achieve the correct balance. Finding the perfect saddle to fit your particular anatomical configuration may take some experimentation. Many women who have experienced saddle discomfort prefer a saddle like the Terry Butterfly.

Adjust the Cleats

Once you have properly aligned the seat height and nose tilt, you must adjust the cleats. Cleats are attached to the bottom of your cycling shoes to help you clip into your pedals securely. Align your feet in a straightforward position, allowing adequate clearance between your heels and the cranks. This is especially important with a pedal system that allows a lot of float. If your feet scrape the cranks during the pedaling stroke, you will lose power and efficiency. The bottoms of your feet should be parallel to the floor with no lateral tilt. If your feet are pronating or supinating, that is, your feet tend to roll in or out, respectively, you may need to replace your shoes or have them professionally shimmed.

Next, the Q needs to be set. The Q refers to the width of the pedals relative to the bottom bracket. I recommend adjusting your cleats to the widest position allowed by your shoes. The objective is to produce the widest stance possible and to put your feet directly under your hips. The greatest combination of power and comfort comes from adjusting the cleats as far to the rear as a standard road shoe will allow. For short, tight circuit races and criteriums, I recommend setting the cleats slightly more forward. Keep in mind that that these adjustments, similar to the fore/aft adjustments, will affect leg angle. Shoes for mountain biking have better ventilation, and I recommend experimenting with a deeper setting that places the cleat slightly behind the ball of the foot, over the first metatarsal joint.

Set the Dimensions of the Cockpit

The cockpit refers to the area where you sit to operate the bike. The setup of the handlebars and the stem varies, depending on whether the angle of the bike frame is shallow for normal roads or steeper for triathlon and time trials. For the road, adjust the brake hoods to provide an ergonomic handhold and a neutral pivot point for braking and shifting. Your elbows should be bent and your wrists should rest gently on the bar. This position is probably not sustainable for long distances; however, it is highly efficient for leveraging power from both the major muscle groups and the core muscles while maintaining a low aero profile (see figure 3.6). Tilt your pelvis forward, hold your back flat, and bend your elbows. Position the stem and tribar assembly so your back can flatten comfortably, which will help increase your endurance and your access to the same major and ancillary muscles used with a road bike.

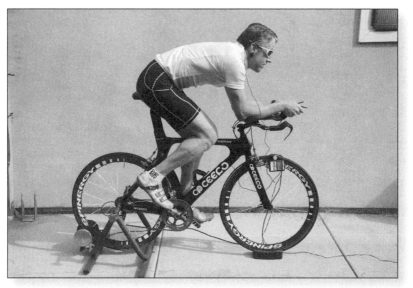

Figure 3.6 Although in the aero position the angles are steeper than those used on a road bike, the overall body position is similar.

The Five Biggest Setup Mistakes Made by Cyclists

A good fit between the cyclist and the bicycle is critical for good performance and injury prevention. Cyclists commonly make a number of mistakes during the initial setup of their bike that steal their power and put stress on their joints and spine. The adjustment features that I most frequently encounter when I fit clients involve the saddle position and the handlebars. Keep in mind that your body will need a little time to adjust to a new position since it is used to compensating in the old one.

Placing the Saddle Too Low

A saddle that is positioned too low does not allow you to access full power from your glutes (your biggest muscles) and your hamstrings. It also puts unnecessary stress on your knees, the weakest point in a cyclist's body.

Tilting the Saddle Upward

When the saddle is tilted upward, it puts an uncomfortable strain on the perineum and the ischial tuberosities (sit bones). It also restricts an important biokinetic chain of events that begins with breathing correctly, tilting your pelvis forward, flattening your back, bending your elbows, and allowing free access to the core. Restriction of this process negatively affects power output.

Adjusting the Saddle Back on the Rails

When the saddle is placed too far back, you trade power and torque for the comfort of an easy chair. Cyclists typically sit with their elbows and wrists locked, which places the center of gravity high. Your elbows should be bent with your wrists poised and tucked in a lower, powerful position that utilizes your core muscles and balances efficiency and aerodynamics.

Flat Pedaling or Dropping the Heels

Pedaling without life in the stroke is a very common mistake that occurs when the saddle is set too low. This is especially prevalent with beginners. Strive for an animated pedal stroke, strongly leading with your toe at the bottom of the stroke. This allows full access to your lower-leg muscles, which exert much-needed pulling power on the backside of the stroke. Correct pedaling provides muscular force through the flexion of the hips.

Placing Brake Hoods Too Low

The hoods must be in a position that allows you to flatten your elbows and rest your hands comfortably. Usually, elevating the hoods allows for greater leverage and control.

The aero bars for the triathlon and time-trial setup should be flat or facing slightly up. Slightly rotating the bars up stabilizes you in the saddle and keeps the saddle nose from drifting forward while you pedal. This also facilitates an aerodynamic posture by closing the open space in front of your chest. Spacers can be added if the steering tube has not been cut too short. You can adjust the length and angle of the stem to improve shoulder and back comfort (see figure 3.6). The stem and bar combination should allow for back comfort in the aero position. Hold your wrists and hands in a neutral position and your elbows at an angle between 95 and 110 degrees.

Careful experimentation is the best method for finding the perfect fit, and it may take a few photo sessions to dial in your bike. Work with a cycling friend to facilitate the process and make it more fun. Be patient and make an effort to feel the effects of every change systematically. When you finish with your fit, take a few minutes to measure the height of the saddle and the reach from the tip of the saddle nose to the center of the bar, and then mark the position of the saddle, rail, bar or hood, and shoe cleats with a strip of tape or color-coded ink to mark your progress.

Training off the Bike

People of various hereditary backgrounds and lifestyles age differently, but some generalities may be drawn. We all lose muscle mass over time, and according to *The Journals of Gerontology, Series A, Biological and Medical Sciences*, muscle biopsies taken from younger and older people indicate that aging causes a significant reduction in the size of fast-twitch or type II muscles fibers, while the slow-twitch or type I muscle fibers are much less affected. As we age, bone density decreases and cartilage wears down and loses its integrity. Our joints stiffen as the synovial fluid loses viscosity and the connective tissue in our ligaments becomes more rigid, limiting our range of motion. Women experience an additional set of issues after menopause. When the anti-inflammatory benefits they once received from estrogen are gone, they may experience joint stiffness or pain and loss of flexibility. Chapter 10 further explores aging in female cyclists.

As the body ages, cell damage progresses. We cannot control some factors that contribute to this damage, such as ultraviolet radiation, free radicals, and genetics, but we can control our behavioral contributions. In his book *It's Better to Believe,* Dr. Ken Cooper says that blood pressure, aerobic capacity, flexibility, and other parameters that change with aging do not decline significantly for people who are physically fit. In fact, they often exhibit better numbers than much younger people who are not fit do.

Flexibility depends on genetics, sex, age, and level of fitness. Whether you are cycling to compete or to improve your aerobic fitness, flexibility training offers several benefits, including greater range of motion, improved posture, relief of muscle soreness and joint stiffness, and reduced risk of injury. Strength training increases metabolism, improves bone density, improves balance and flexibility, reduces the probability of injury, and develops lean muscle, strength, and endurance. Combining flexibility and strength training ensures that your body is prepared to train on the bicycle with better and faster results. Let's start with flexibility.

TYPES OF FLEXIBILITY

Flexibility is one of the many components of fitness. Yoga is an example of *passive flexibility*, or using your body weight and gravity to increase the depth of the stretch while holding limbs or other parts of your body in extended positions. *Active flexibility* uses the tension of the muscle opposite to the one being stretched when assuming and holding extended positions. I use a combination of the two types in my stretching routine and often use a fitness ball to increase the stretch and to strengthen core muscles.

Flexibility can be obtained a number of ways, but the most effective means is with a comprehensive stretching program. Stretching is a bit like a religion. Some of us are fervent believers, starting or ending each day with our favorite stretching regimens. Some cyclists give it lip service, performing perfunctory toe touches and a few ballistic (bouncing) stretches of the hamstrings and quadriceps before a run or a bike ride. Others abstain from stretching completely, thinking it a pointless and time-consuming inconvenience. Jay Blahnik, author of *Full-Body Flexibility*, says that "[flexibility] is a reward you can feel every day."

Stretching is a prerequisite for flexibility, and flexibility is a prerequisite for avoiding injury. Once you have experienced a regular stretching program, the physical and mental benefits will quickly become apparent. Flexibility improves balance and extends and maintains your range of motion. It also relieves chronic pain, reduces stress, increases energy, and improves circulation, mental focus, and posture. "Stretching is about learning to relax in a comfortable, individual way. It allows you to get back in touch with the way you feel," says Bob Anderson, author of *Stretching in the Office*.

Although the benefits are real, some people lack the discipline to stretch on their own. If you are one of these people, consider joining a yoga class, which offers a structured venue for stretching and building core strength. Many gyms offer classes for all levels of ability, and you will not find a more supportive group than the community of yoga practitioners. For those who are better disciplined, I offer a program that is guaranteed to improve your flexibility and core strength. I will present a large number of stretches and exercises here that a person would find it difficult to incorporate into a daily routine. However, a

Cycling for Life

Wayne Stetina

Wayne Stetina, a former Olympic teammate and longtime friend, has been racing since he was 9 years old. As a junior competitor, he medaled several times at the 1970 and 1971 Nationals in road and track. At the elite level, Wayne competed with the U.S national road team for 17 years, and he served as a member of U.S. cycling teams for three Olympic Games and four World Championships. His many achievements in the sport include taking gold in the time trial at the Pan American Games in 1975 and winning the Red Zinger Classic in 1977. He retired from full-time competition in 1985 to work for Shimano. Wayne continues to race at the masters level and holds six national road titles and two national criterium titles.

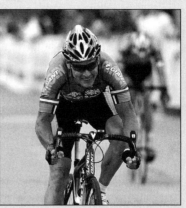

Wayne Stetina's winning sprint at the masters national criterium championship in 2008.

At 55 years of age, Wayne finds that he cannot recover as quickly from consecutive days of hard, sustained efforts on the bike, especially when climbing in the mountains or doing hill repeats. He needs one or two easy days following a hard ride; if he rides hard for two consecutive days, he may need up to a week of easy days to recover completely. By consistently working his core muscles, riding gently, and doing some kind of workout daily, Wayne dropped some weight, which made it easier for him to climb hills. He now races about once a month and tries to maintain a top level of fitness.

"I want to stay fit so that I can train with the top-level pros doing four- to six-hour rides with lots of climbing at their training camp," says Stetina. "My nephew Peter (son of former Olympian Dale Stetina) is on the Garmin team, and I got to train with the entire team, climbing through the hills around Solvang in January before the Tour of California in 2009." Racing is a family tradition for the Stetinas, Roy, Wayne, and Dale's father, who was a top road racer in his youth. Wayne credits his father as being his only coach when he began racing as a junior.

selection of strengthening and stretching exercises that vary from day to day will make the number more manageable. For example, a selection of at least four to five core exercises should be done each day. The weight training should be limited to 3 days per week for a period of 30 minutes each, and you will be more actively involved with this during the off-season than when your cycling mileage begins to peak.

STRETCHING FOR FLEXIBILITY

Everything you do off the bike affects what happens on the bike. Instead of thinking of stretching as something you must do each day, think of it as something to look forward to. This practice will make you a better cyclist. The best way to make a stretching regimen stick is to hit the floor after you awake each morning and run through a brief, ancillary core routine. This gets the blood flowing and lubricates the joints before you start to stretch the major muscle groups. In my experience, once you see the positive effects of flexibility for your cycling performance, you will increase the duration and frequency of your core and flexibility workouts. Think of these workouts as money in the bank for cycling that is more powerful and efficient.

This set of exercises and stretches will peak your athleticism, boost your performance, and protect you against injury. You will notice the quality of your sleep improving with workouts of just 15 minutes per day. The first series of four core exercises gets the blood flowing and prepares the body for stretching. Breathe deeply, filling the chest cavity with air until the abdomen completely contracts, then exhale, expelling every bit of air out of your body. The heart pumps oxygenated blood into the stretched muscles and synovial fluid into the joints, vastly improving the quality of the stretch. This technique engages the parasympathetic nervous system for stretching that is deeper and strength training that is more controlled. Practice each stretch with a forceful and audible exhalation.

Foam Roller Across the Spine

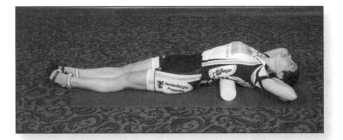

Figure 4.1 Foam roller across the spine.

Most of our daily activities, such as riding a bike and sitting in front of a computer, reduce mobility of the spine and cause us to bend our backs in an unhealthy, curving posture. The roller works the spine in small sections, counterstretching it to correct the stooped posture caused by long hours in the saddle (figure 4.1). It also opens the intercostal muscles in the chest, that is, the muscles lying over and under the ribs that contract and expand the chest cavity, which facilitates breathing, promotes blood flow, transfers synovial fluids, and warms up the body. Work the middle of the spine (vertebrae T6 to T12). Beginners should do 10 seconds per 2-inch (5 cm) section, and those who are more advanced should do two sets. When you are finished, dismount by rolling off to the side. Avoid abdominal crunches, which can displace vertebrae, during the dismount.

Recumbent Cycling

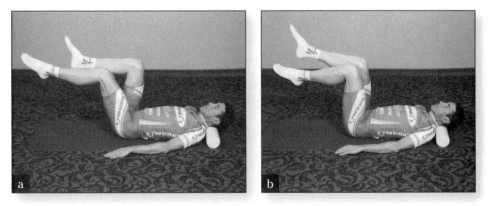

Figure 4.2 Recumbent cycling.

Lie on a mat on your back in the recumbent position, and then kick your hips with your heels to break up lactic acid and muscle adhesions in your quadriceps (figure 4.2). From this initial warm-up position, extend your legs, point your toes, and make small, tight circles with your feet. Beginners should do 15 repetitions on each leg, and those who are more advanced should do 50.

Recumbent Oblique Cycling

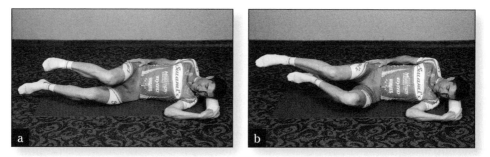

Figure 4.3   Recumbent oblique cycling.

Use the same routine described in the previous exercise, but perform first on one side, then the other. Beginners should do 5 to 10 repetitions on each side, and those who are more advanced should do 25 to 30 repetitions on each side (figure 4.3).

Recumbent Warm-Up and Stretch for Adductor and Abductor Muscles

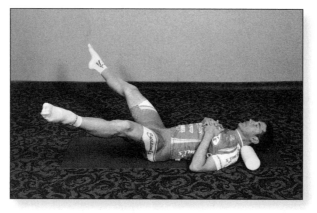

Figure 4.4   Recumbent warm-up and stretch for adductor and abductor muscles.

To perform the stretch, lie on your back and elevate your legs. Hold your knees together, straighten your legs, point your toes in slightly, and then spread your legs as wide apart as possible (figure 4.4). Hold them apart for a second before returning to the starting position. Beginners should do five repetitions, and those who are more advanced should do 20 repetitions.

Stretch for Hip and Groin Muscles

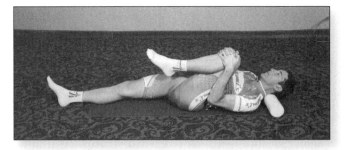

Figure 4.5   Stretch for hip and groin muscles.

Tightness in the groin, psoas (one of the hip flexors), and hip muscles reduces core flexibility and range of motion. To perform the stretch, lie flat on your back and stretch your legs straight out. Keep one leg flat on the floor, and pull the knee of your other leg toward your chest (figure 4.5). Extend the leg on the floor as you inhale, and pull the other knee in closer as you exhale. Each repetition should bring the knee a little closer to the chest. You will have achieved maximum flexibility when you can touch each knee to your chest. Beginners should do four or five repetitions on each leg, and those who are more advanced should do 8 to 10 repetitions.

Stretch for the Adductor, Pectineus, and Gracilis Muscles

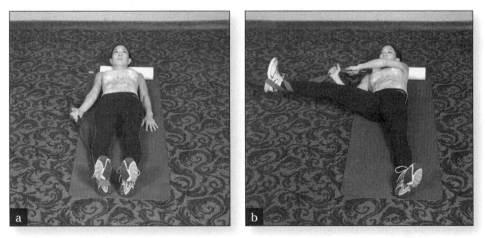

Figure 4.6   Stretch for the adductor, pectineus, and gracilis muscles.

The muscles of the inner thigh become tight without concentric contraction. To perform the stretch, attach a strap around your foot and under your calf for knee support. Flexing your foot, draw your leg away from your body in a low arc (figure 4.6). Exhale as you extend your leg. Beginners should do four to six repetitions on each leg, and those who are more advanced should do 8 to 10 repetitions on each leg.

Stretch for the Iliotibial Bands

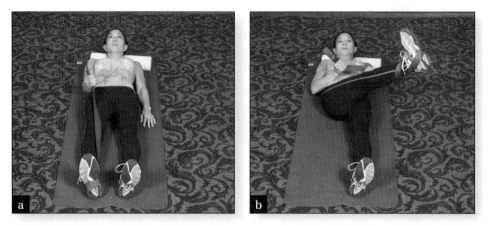

Figure 4.7 Stretch for the iliotibial bands.

Tightness in the iliotibial (IT) bands, which run from the hip to the knee, is common for cyclists and runners who do not stretch regularly. During cycling, the legs track away from the body rather than linearly along the forward vector, exerting extra pressure on the knee. This stretch can help you save your knees. To perform the stretch, wrap a strap around your foot and under your ankle and calf to support your knee joint. Lie with your hips and shoulders flat on the floor, and then bring your leg across the body at a low angle, pointing your toes at the ceiling (figure 4.7). Hold the stretch for one long exhalation, and then return your leg to the forward position. Beginners should limit their practice to four to six repetitions. Advanced athletes can repeat this stretch 8 to 10 times.

Active Stretch for External Hip Rotators

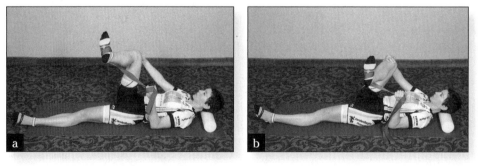

Figure 4.8 Active stretch for external hip rotators.

Contracture and reduced range of motion of the external hip rotators can make your knees splay, which causes a loss of power during the most powerful arc of the pedaling stroke. Splayed knees also create poor aerodynamics and decrease stability, especially during descents. To perform the stretch, lie on your back, and wrap a strap around your foot. Bend your knee to a 90-degree angle, then use the strap to pull your knee across your body (figure 4.8). Do this stretch before aerobic activity. Beginners should do four to six repetitions on each leg, and those who are more advanced should do 8 to 10 repetitions per side.

Passive Stretch for External Hip Rotators

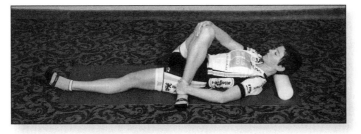

Figure 4.9 Passive stretch for external hip rotators.

This passive stretch is essentially similar to the preceding version but eliminates the repetitions. It loosens up the external hip rotators to improve alignment of the legs and engagement of the gluteal muscles. To perform this stretch, lie on your back with one leg outstretched and the other leg bent. Place the foot of your bent leg flat on the ground and pull the other leg over to rest on the quadriceps of the bent leg. Reach up and grasp your bent leg behind the knee and then pull back gently to move your straightened leg perpendicular to the body (figure 4.9). If you are not yet flexible enough for this option, simply place the strap around the foot and ankle of your outstretched leg and use it to move into the position. Gradually intensify the pressure. Do this stretch after your primary aerobic activity. Beginners should hold the stretch for 15 seconds, and those who are more advanced should hold it for 45 seconds.

Passive Bilateral Stretch for Piriformis Muscles

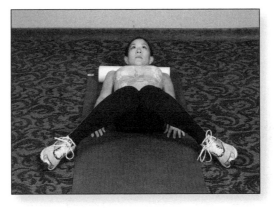

Figure 4.10 Passive bilateral stretch for piriformis muscles.

This exercise, along with the groin rock and groin release, is one of a series of three stretches that open up the hips and groin, increasing fluidity of the gluteal muscles, utilization of the stabilizing core muscles, and optimization of the parasympathetic breathing technique. Bilaterally and passively stretching the piriformis muscles externally opens these hip rotators and helps them function more efficiently. To perform the stretch, lie on your back with your knees bent. Hold your feet as far apart as possible and bring your knees together very slightly (figure 4.10). Beginners should hold this stretch for 15 seconds, while those who are more advanced may hold it for 30 seconds.

Groin Rock

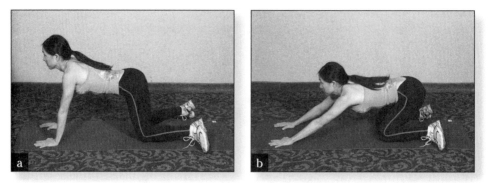

Figure 4.11 Groin rock.

This exercise is the second in a series of three stretches that open up the hips and groin. Following the piriformis stretch, the groin rock switches from front to back, opening the groin and lower back to facilitate a full aerodynamic tuck. To perform the stretch, assume a position with the knees on the floor and the torso held up with straightened arms (figure 4.11). Release into a forward position and then move back and forth between the two positions for 5 to 7 repetitions.

Groin Release

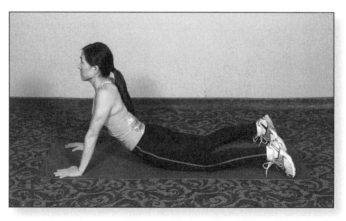

Figure 4.12 Groin release.

This exercise is the third in a series of three stretches that open up the hips and groin. It breaks up lactic acid accumulated in the muscles. To perform the stretch, assume a position with the hips on the floor and the torso held up with straightened arms (figure 4.12). Beginners should hold the stretch for 5 seconds with five or six repetitions, while those who are more advanced may hold it for 5 seconds with 8 to 10 repetitions.

Stretch for Hamstrings

Tightness in the hamstrings severely limits your ability to bend forward at the hips. This condition pulls the pelvis into a posterior tilt, making it more difficult to flatten your back and sit low on the bike. Tight hamstrings also rob your legs of horsepower. To perform this stretch, lie down flat on your back with your legs straight. Place a rolled-up towel in the small of your back and position one foot against the wall to improve stability if necessary. Anchor the strap around the ball of the other foot and pull it back slowly keeping the leg straight. Repeat with the other leg. Perform this stretch both before and after your ride or run. Beginners should do four to six repetitions, holding each stretch for one long exhalation. Those who are more advanced should perform 8 to 10 repetitions.

Active Stretch for Quadriceps

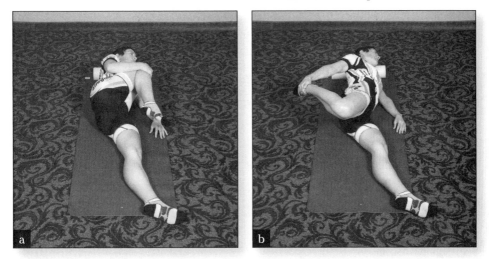

Figure 4.13   Active stretch for quadriceps.

A good range of motion for these primary muscles will help your knees track smoothly and will improve your follow-through during the power portion of your cycling stroke. Stretch your quadriceps after a ride to avoid stagnation and slow legs the next day. To perform this stretch, lie on the floor on your side and bend the knee of your top leg toward your chest. Grasp your top foot and pull it back, then allow the knee to return to your chest (figure 4.13). Hold the leg on the floor straight and remain on your side. Beginners should do four to six repetitions, and those who are more advanced should do 8 to 10 repetitions. After completing the quadriceps stretch, stretch the outer hip by bringing your knee forward against your chest. Flex your foot as you push your knee down and place your leg on top of the other. Combine this stretch with the following version for optimal results.

Passive Stretch for Quadriceps

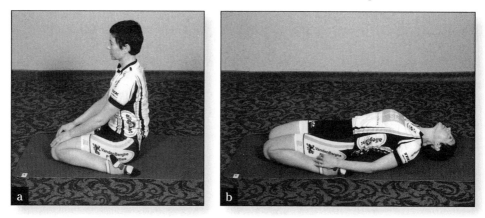

Figure 4.14 Passive stretch for quadriceps.

Only advanced athletes should perform this stretch. To perform this stretch, sit on the floor with your knees bent beneath you and slowly lean back until your head and upper back are resting on the floor. Proceed gently and do not force yourself to deepen the stretch (figure 4.14). Combine this stretch with the active version described in the previous exercise for optimal results.

Modified Push-Up

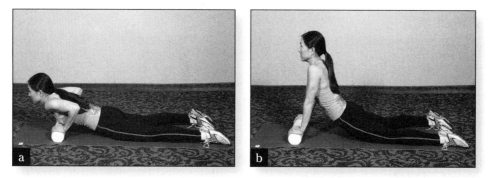

Figure 4.15 Modified push-up.

This stretch improves flexibility of the lower back and stretches the vertical muscles of the back. It will stretch the erector spinae muscles in the back and will strengthen the muscles of the lower back. To perform this stretch, lie face down on the floor. Keeping your lower body dormant, elevate your body from the waist up by straightening your arms (figure 4.15). Beginners should do three to five repetitions, holding each for an extended exhalation of five seconds. Those who are more advanced should perform five to eight repetitions, following the same technique.

Hanging Stretch

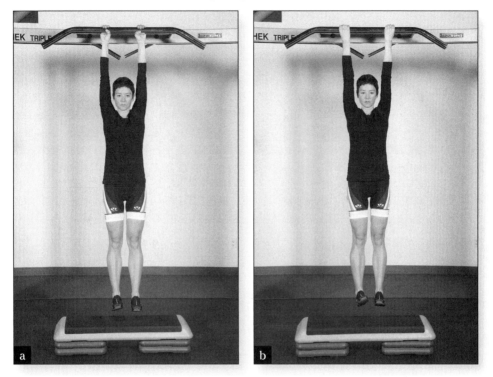

Figure 4.16 Hanging stretch.

This stretch also focuses on upper-body flexibility and stretches out the spine. It requires a chin-up bar. To perform the stretch, hang from the bar holding your hands in both over- and underhanded positions to work different muscles (figure 4.16). Beginners should hang for 15 seconds in each position, and those who are more advanced should hang for 30 seconds.

Bent-Knee Calf Stretch

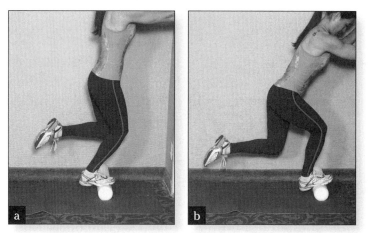

Figure 4.17 Bent-knee calf stretch.

Stand on a step or platform and allow your heel to hang off the edge, and bend your knee. Slowly drop one of your heels as far as it will go and then switch feet (figure 4.17). This is another isolated, passive stretch that works the calf muscles. Beginners should hold the stretch for 15 seconds on each side, and those who are more advanced should hold it for 30 seconds.

Stretch for Upper Trapezius Muscles

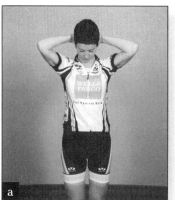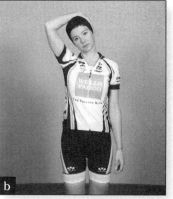

Figure 4.18 Stretch for upper trapezius muscles.

This stretch focuses on upper-body flexibility, one of the most common problem areas for cyclists. The objective is to balance and strengthen the posterior thoracic muscles, such as the trapezius, levator scapulae, and rhomboids, to increase biomechanical and aerodynamic efficiency. Do this stretch before and immediately after a long ride. To perform the stretch, tuck your chin, find the bony lump at the base of your skull, hold that area, and pull gently to one side (figure 4.18). After several seconds, lift the opposite shoulder. Do three to five repetitions on each side for five seconds (beginner and advanced).

Straight-Leg Calf Stretch

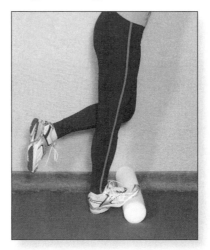

Figure 4.19 Straight-leg calf stretch.

Stand on a step or platform and allow your heel to hang off the edge. Face straight ahead. Holding your leg straight, slowly drop one of your heels as low as it will go and then switch feet. This is an isolated, passive stretch (figure 4.19). Beginners should hold the stretch for 15 seconds. Those who are more advanced should hold it for 30 seconds.

Side Stretch on a Ball

When done correctly, this stretch opens the section of the body between the attachment of the IT bands and the armpit and loosens the lower back. Stand and brace your body, placing your legs in a wide stance. Bend at the waist to lie on your side over the top of an exercise ball. Extend the arm that is nearest the ball and hold the upper wrist of that arm with your other hand. Extend your top leg and place it in alignment with your upper body. Repeat on the other side. Beginners should hold the stretch for 30 seconds once on each side, while experts may stretch twice on each side for the same amount of time.

Body-Weight Press

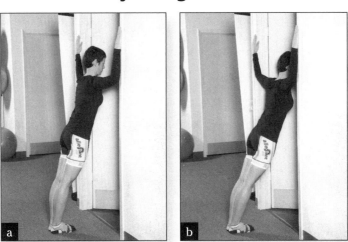

Figure 4.20 Body-weight press.

This stretch focuses on upper-body flexibility. When done deeply and correctly, it opens the intercostal muscles in the chest for more efficient breathing. To perform the stretch, stand in a doorway holding your arms at shoulder level and your forearms against the doorjamb. Lean forward through into the open space, allowing your body weight to open up the chest muscles (figure 4.20). All levels of athletes should do three repetitions of 10 to 15 seconds. Perform this stretch after your ride.

Bilaterial Stretch for the Pectoralis Minor

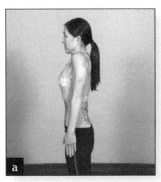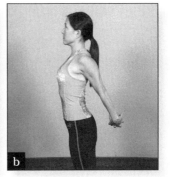

Figure 4.21 Bilateral stretch for pectoralis minor.

This stretch focuses on upper-body flexibility. Deep shrugs open the chest muscles for more relaxed breathing during high output efforts. Do this stretch while standing. To perform the stretch, shrug your shoulders deeply and then pull them back, clasping your hands behind your back and squeezing your shoulder blades together (figure 4.21). Athletes of all levels should hold the position for the duration of six deep breaths. This stretch is excellent for after a ride.

STRENGTHENING A FLEXIBLE BODY

With an acceptable level of flexibility, the body is better prepared for resistance training. Strength training does much more than fortify targeted muscle groups. It increases metabolism so that the body burns more calories in a 24-hour period; it increases bone density, reducing the risk for fractures; and it increases muscle mass, making the body leaner, stronger, and more resilient. A well-rounded program strengthens the muscles, joints, tendons, and ligaments to improve flexibility, balance, and joint stability. Studies have shown that strength training promotes positive changes in blood cholesterol and decreases systolic and diastolic blood pressure. Our mobility, independence, and ability to enjoy life as we age are enhanced by strength training. Best of all, increased strength and flexibility make for better athletes.

Before beginning strength training, engage the body in a warm-up routine. I recommend 15 minutes on the bike trainer followed by the stretches previously mentioned. Muscles remember the last activity they performed, so establish neurological pathways to maximize muscle memory by cooling down with another 15 minutes on the trainer after strength training. Use good form. Stop if fatigue causes your form to deteriorate. How you schedule your workouts depends on your individual needs and time constraints.

The following strength exercises have been developed specifically for cyclists. You should notice an improvement in your power and endurance within weeks of starting this program.

Reclining Roll on a Ball

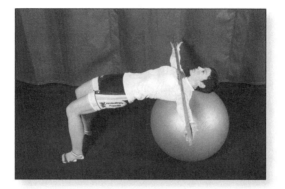

Figure 4.22 Reclining roll on a ball.

This exercise strengthens the abdominal and erector spinae muscles, which are important for climbing. Use a mirror and a spotter to check your form. Use the ball to support your head as you focus on the ceiling. Balance a long pole on your chest, holding your hands open and facing up (figure 4.22). Raise your buttocks, contract your glutes, and walk 10 inches (25 cm) to one side and then to the other while supporting the pole.

Hip Extension and Knee Flexion on a Ball

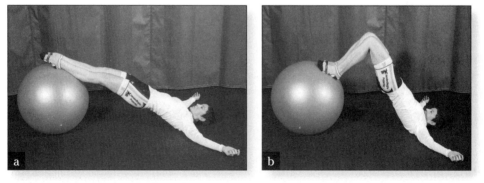

Figure 4.23 Hip extension and knee flexion on a ball.

This two-step exercise strengthens the core and gluteal muscles. Lie over the ball on your back, bracing your feet against the ball. Straighten your back, elevate your hips and torso, and stretch your arms out to the sides. Your body should form a straight line from knees to shoulders. Use your feet to draw the ball toward your body. Bend your knees until your feet are flat on the ball and your body forms a steep, inverted *V* (figure 4.23). Beginners should do two to four repetitions per set, and those who are more advanced should do six to eight repetitions per set.

Press With Corrective Holistic Exercise Kinesiology (CHEK)

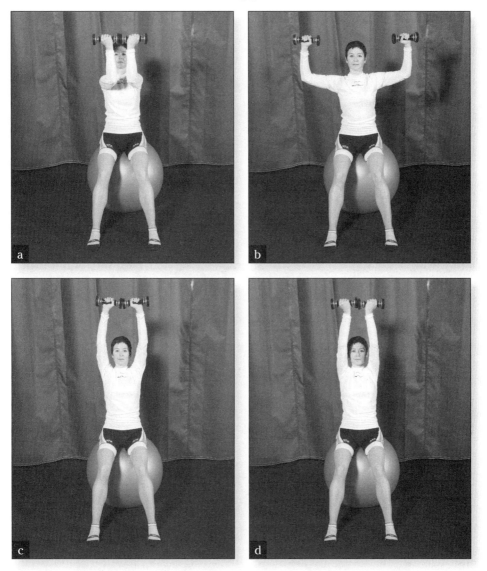

Figure 4.24 CHEK press.

Cyclists need very specific exercises for inversion, rotation, and extension to improve strength and range of motion for the upper body while staying lean. This press has four parts. Using good posture, hold a dumbbell in each hand and sit on the ball, Bend your elbows to form a 90-degree angle. Maintaining good posture, squeeze your shoulder blades together and bring your arms as far back as you can. Next, raise your arms over your head with the palms facing forward. Invert the weights so your palms are facing backward and return your arms to the starting position (figure 4.24). Repeat the series 8 to 12 times per set, performing two or three sets. Start with light weights, and rest for 30 seconds between sets.

Squat, Push, and Press

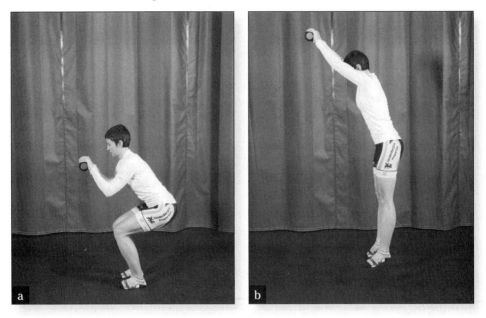

Figure 4.25 Squat, push, and press.

This explosive plyometric drill is specific to cycling since it supercharges fast-twitch muscle fibers. Start by holding light weights in each hand. Place your feet shoulder-width apart, pointing your toes out slightly, and squat, holding your knees out. Push the weights straight up over your head with an explosive movement, and stretch your muscles at the top (figure 4.25). Bring the weights back down and hold them at chest level. Do this exercise in front of a mirror to check your form. Repeat the cycle 8 to 12 times per set, and do two or three sets, allowing a full minute for recovery between sets.

Prone Elevation of Trunk and Hips (Superman)

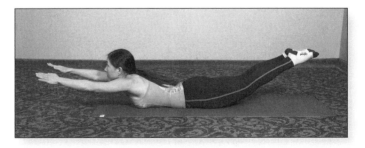

Figure 4.26 Prone elevation of trunk and hips (Superman).

Lie face down on the floor, and then simultaneously elevate your legs, torso, arms, and head (figure 4.26). Beginners should start with three repetitions of 15 seconds, resting for 15 seconds in between. Those who are more advanced should do six repetitions of 30 to 45 seconds, resting for 30 seconds in between.

Howard Counter Curve (Passive)

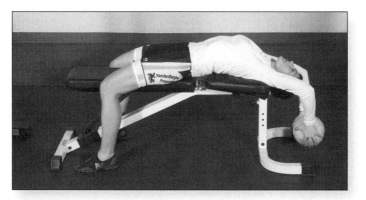

Figure 4.27 Howard counter curve (passive).

This exercise stretches, strengthens, and flattens the back to correct hours of holding a lordotic curve in the saddle. Use a bench or a ball and a weight that is light enough to allow for full range of motion. Grasp the weight with both hands and hold it behind your head (figure 4.27). Beginners should hold the stretch for 15 seconds. Those who are more advanced should do the stretch twice for 30 seconds.

Walking Forward and Backward Lunges

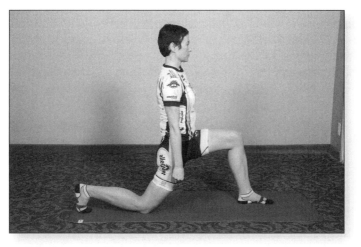

Figure 4.28 Walking forward and backward lunges.

Keep your upper body erect, your head straight, and your eyes forward. Step forward using KOPS alignment (knee over pedal spindle), and return to a neutral position (figure 4.28). Step back with the same leg, using the KOPS alignment again. If balance is an issue, try resting a pole on your shoulders. You might also try some light hand weights. Beginners should do a single set of lunges, walking forward. Those who are more advanced should do two sets of 8 to 12 lunges, walking forward and backward and resting for 60 seconds between sets.

Hamstring Rotations

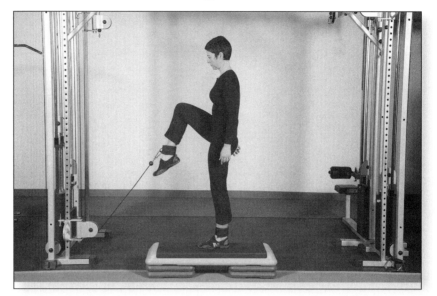

Figure 4.29 Hamstring rotations.

Use this exercise as your primary strength builder for the hamstrings. Use a lower pulley machine and ankle straps to replicate the exact motor action of pedaling (figure 4.29). Elevate your supporting leg with a flat platform, such as a step, so that you can follow through the stroke with dominant planter flexion (your toe leads down at the bottom of the stroke). Alternate your legs to stretch the hip flexors. Beginners should do one set of six repetitions on each side using 10 to 20 pounds (4.5-9 kg). Those who are more advanced should do two sets of 8 to 12 repetitions using 20 to 40 pounds (9-18 kg).

Hip-Flexor Rotations

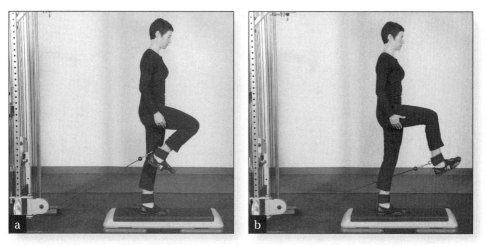

Figure 4.30   Hip-flexor rotations.

This exercise works in tandem with the hamstring rotation. Using the same setup as the in previous exercise, face away from the machine and replicate a pedal stroke (figure 4.30). Since you will be alternating legs, you do not need to rest between sets. Each set of hip-flexor rotations on one leg should be followed by a set on the other leg.

Strengthening the Adductor and Abductor Muscles

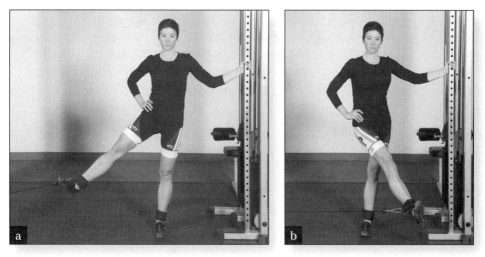

Figure 4.31   Strengthening the adductor and abductor muscles.

You may do this exercise with either an adductor and abductor machine or a lower pulley and an ankle strap. Working one leg at a time, flex it and pull it straight across and in front of the other (figure 4.31). You can also use ankle weights while lying on one side. Do 8 to 10 repetitions per set and two or three sets per leg.

Calf Extensions and Raises

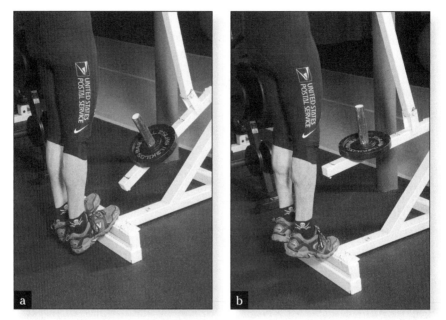

Figure 4.32 Calf extensions and raises.

Use a calf machine for this exercise. Start with little or no weight. Holding your shoulders under the pads and the ball of each foot on the platform, allow your heels to drop below the level of the platform, keeping your posture erect. This extends the muscles. Next, raise your heels above the level of the platform, pushing your shoulders against the pads as you elevate your body (figure 4.32). Repeat this sequence 12 times per set for two sets, resting for 30 seconds between sets. Increase the weight in small increments as your calves strengthen and as you become more comfortable with the exercise.

Leg Press

This press builds serious strength in the gluteal muscles. Sit at a leg-press machine, place your feet against the platform, and straighten your legs to press the weight up. Avoid using heavy weights and going too deep on the release. Keep your bottom on the seat and your feet flat on the platform and evenly spaced. Beginners should do 10 repetitions for a single set, and those who are more advanced should do 12 to 15 repetitions per set.

Leg Extensions

Working one leg at a time on a pulley machine, extend your lower leg until it is straight. Hold the stretch for a count, and then lower your leg. Start without any weight on the pulley, then gradually add resistance, bar by bar. Repeat sets, holding your toes both out and in. Do 10 to 12 repetitions per set and two or three sets.

Flexibility and performance are vastly improved by stretching and by doing weight training. You must observe good form. If fatigue begins to affect your form, stop and move on to the next exercise. Performing stretches with incorrect form can result in injury. If you are uncertain about how to operate a particular machine, please ask a trainer at your gym to demonstrate the correct technique.

Training Indoors on the Bike

Inclement weather, time constraints, or other issues may compel you to train indoors occasionally or frequently, depending on your geographic location or lifestyle. Indoor training eliminates a number of concerns from your routine, including traffic, road hazards that could puncture tires, and remembering to bring enough food or water for the ride home.

However, getting good workouts on an indoor trainer requires discipline and time. The first couple of weeks of indoor training can be somewhat daunting since pedaling in one spot is not terribly exciting. If you can get past that initial phase, you will begin to enjoy your indoor rides more and find them more valuable. I recommend a varied workout with different levels of intensity that lasts no more than one hour. If you need more variety, you can use different pieces of equipment and computerized systems that can measure your output and provide interactive challenges to make the experience more fun.

BICYCLE ROLLERS

Bicycle rollers have been around for a long time. Charles "Mile-a-Minute" Murphy was a six-day racer at Madison Square Garden in the 1890s. He claimed the land-speed record on a bicycle when he traveled 60 miles (97 km) per hour while being paced by the Long Island Express. Wooden planks were placed over the ties so that he could ride in the slipstream of the train. Murphy also designed wooden rollers to ride on as an indoor-training tool and staged roller competitions at Keith's Orpheum, a popular vaudeville circus show. He challenged African-American racing star, Major Taylor, to duels in various cities as part of the show. Murphy's presentation was very similar to the Rollapaluza roller races held in Great Britain today. In Britain in the 1940s and '50s, roller races were held at cinemas before film showings and were staged at dance halls between dances. Rollapaluza is committed to reviving this time-honored sport. In 2008, they ran 75 roller races with more than 6,000 contestants.

Rollers consist of three drums attached to a frame, one for the front wheel and two for the rear wheel. A belt connects one of the rear drums to the front drum, which allows the front wheel of a bicycle placed on the rollers to spin when you pedal. The front drum adjusts to fit the bicycle's wheelbase and usually sits slightly ahead of the hub of the front wheel. Drums can be made of wood, aluminum, or plastic, but aluminum is the best material for avoiding distortion over time. The frames are composed of welded steel or extruded aluminum, the latter of which is much lighter for transporting.

Riding on rollers helps improve bike-handling skills. The challenge is to maintain balance on the rollers while cycling, which requires a smooth pedaling stroke. Some systems have drums with indentations that help keep the bike from drifting off. You can also attach a fork stand for sprints out of the saddle or single-leg drills, or to eliminate balance issues altogether during a workout. Drums come in a range of sizes. Smaller diameters create greater resistance due to friction from bearings and tires. If you are uncertain about how much resistance you want, I recommend the popular 4.5-inch (11-cm) diameter drums. If needed, increase resistance by adding a flywheel or a headwind fan.

Quality aluminum rollers can be purchased for $300 USD or more. Some innovative systems, such as the Rocking Rollers, have been developed to prevent you from drifting off the rollers. You can ride out of the saddle, assume an aero position, or mash the pedals with the manufacturer's guarantee that you will not ride off these rollers. They have a magnet enclosed by a plastic swivel-arm that is located next to a flywheel. You can rotate the arm in or out of engagement with the face of the flywheel to change the resistance level. They retail for nearly $800 USD.

REAR-WHEEL TRAINERS

With this type of trainer, the rear hub of your bicycle is mounted on the unit and the front wheel sits on a riser so that the bike is level and the front wheel is stationary. Some units have integrated fork stands to elevate and stabilize the front of the bike. Some trainers use magnetoresistance, and others use fluid or flywheels for resistance. Most magnetic trainers are driven by the tire, but other models are driven by the rim. Basic versions of rear-wheel trainers run from $80 to $200 USD, getting more expensive as features are added.

You can also purchase rear-wheel training systems that are integrated with a computer, such as the Tacx i-Magic, PowerTap products, or my personal favorite, the CompuTrainer. Computer-integrated rear-wheel trainers measure the effects

One-Hour Trainer Workout

1. Warm up for 15 minutes with 10 hypoxic intervals of 15 seconds. At the beginning of every 60-second interval, hold your breath for 15 seconds while pedaling. Gradually build your rpm (between 80 and 100).

2. Do six single-leg drills of 30 seconds on each leg (see chapter 8 for single-leg drills).

3. Do the following ladder workout for 15 minutes (see pages 75-79 for training zones):
   - Work for 15 seconds in zone 3 and rest for 15 seconds.
   - Work for 30 seconds in zone 3 and rest for 30 seconds.
   - Work for 45 seconds in zone 4 and rest for 45 seconds.
   - Work for 30 seconds in zone 3. Increase your rpm by 10 percent.
   - Work for 15 seconds in zone 3. Increase your rpm again by 10 percent.

4. Do 15 minutes of $\dot{V}O_2$max intervals:
   - Work for 60 seconds in zone 4. Repeat the cycle six times with one minute of active recovery in between.
   - Spin pedals for three minutes at 110 rpm.
   - Work for 20 seconds in zone 5. Repeat the cycle six times with 10 seconds of recovery between intervals.

5. Do a recovery spin at 110 rpm for 10 minutes.

6. Work for 10 minutes in the high end of zone 3 (big chain ring) at 50 rpm.

7. Work for 5 minutes, moving from zone 3 to 2. Gradually decrease your rpm from 100 to 60.

Coach Jay's Little Big Horn Workout

Spin classes are available that let you set up your road bike on your own trainer and riser. If you're ever in Billings, Montana, in the middle of winter, Coach Jay Marschall holds a weekly spin class in a local bike shop that defines the ideal indoor-training session. Coach Jay conducted these workouts in Atlanta and Boston before moving to Billings, and he really knows how to throw a training party. The classes, which realistically replicate outdoor riding, are always sold out, attracting famous cyclists and triathletes from all over the American West.

Coach Jay prefers that you bring your own bike, trainer, and mat. However, since these workouts are conducted at a bike shop, he can provide a trainer and a bike if you ask in advance. The powerful hour and a half of cycling includes Coach Jay's voice instruction, videos of racing footage projected on a large overhead screen, supportive camaraderie, and a competitive environment that will bring out your off-season form. After the hammer session, join everyone for pizza and beer at the favorite local spot. The experience will become your best excuse for returning the following week. Look around your area for a bike shop that has a similar program.

of power both indoors and outdoors and help you train through cutting-edge programs that offer greater depth of experience and workouts with more variety. Trainers help you monitor and compare the values of power and heart rate and let you perform stroke analyses on the road. Indoor devices with an electronic load control, such as the CompuTrainer, simulate the degree of slope for any course in the world. You can add resistance components like headwind and tailwind to challenge your speed. Pennsylvanian Ken Glah trained for the Ironman competition in New Zealand in the dead of winter, using his CompuTrainer to simulate the tough 112-mile (180 km) bike course. He won the overall race without any outdoor training. Another advantage of indoor simulators is their rapid acquisition of data and subsequent in-depth analysis. You can analyze your pedal stroke for efficiency, measure the power the stroke generates, and see the results on the screen.

Don't scoff at the idea of spending hours on a trainer. The best simulators have 3-D pacers that can be activated in several ways: They can ride in front of you for drafting, ride to the side, or sprint away from you, compelling you to give chase. As in an interactive video game, you can change the role of the pacers at will, inflicting pain or joy to match what you want out of the workout. You watch your progress relative to the pacers on the screen as you race along the course. Some systems, including the CompuTrainer, allow multiple cyclists on their trainers to interact and compete on the same system. The CompuTrainer comes with established bike courses from popular races, and you can download courses from your GPS to add routes that you like for training or sharing with friends.

STATIONARY BIKES

Stationary bicycles are typically used in spin classes and run anywhere from $120 to $5,000 USD, depending on the bells and whistles. You can buy recumbents that are relatively inexpensive or uprights with displays that indicate the speed, distance, time, and calories burned. CatEye has a number of computerized products, including the GameBike Pro Exercise Bike, an interactive system that works with the PlayStation or Xbox. You simply plug it in and play. You control every movement on the screen with your motion on the bike, such as steering, turning, speed, strategy, and more. I've been told that the time just flies with this system. You may be surprised to realize that you have spent hours pedaling.

Spin classes provide fun and challenging workouts on stationary bikes and are great if you're short on time. Most fitness clubs include spin classes in the membership fee, and larger facilities offer these classes many times during the day, including early mornings, lunch hour, and evenings to cater to working members. Particular classes may have a focus, such as interval training, high-cadence cycling, simulated road rides, climbing workouts, and all-terrain rides. You may ride to music and videos. Targets for heart rates are often suggested. A good instructor motivates you to push the limits of your endurance and to get the most out of the experience. You will quickly learn who the best instructors are.

Spin classes give you a good cardio workout, but they are no replacement for being on the road outdoors. The flywheel mechanism adds momentum to the backstroke of your pedal motion, reducing its effectiveness relative to the same motion on a regular bicycle. For indoor training, I prefer rollers to a rear-wheel trainer, and training on a stationary bike should be a last resort. If you like the concept of spinning in a group, try to find a spin class that lets you bring in your own bicycle.

INDOOR CYCLING TRACKS

If your city has an indoor velodrome, you may have another option for indoor training. In the late 19th and early 20th centuries, track racing was more popular than baseball. Many tracks had standing room only, and six-day races were attended enthusiastically. Cycling stars, such as Major Taylor, Eddie Bald, Floyd McFarland, Alf Goullet, Jimmy Walthour, and Alf Letourneur, stormed the ovals to cheering crowds, making between $500 and $1,000 USD a day. Interest in track racing waned with the emergence of the automobile and the economic hardships of the Great Depression.

Indoor cycling is enjoying a resurgence in popularity around the world, and new indoor velodromes are popping up in cities all over, such as Boulder, Colorado; Burnaby, British Colombia (near Vancouver); and London, Ontario, in eastern Canada. Plans are being made and funds are being raised for new indoor velodromes in Chicago, Illinois; Cleveland, Ohio; Broomfield, Colorado; Las Vegas, Nevada; and Roubaix, France, among other cities. Australia has several indoor velodromes, and New Zealand has a new one as well. A velodrome was built in Hong Kong for the Beijing Olympics, and one opened in Carson, California (near Los Angeles) in 2004. Indoor velodromes are more common in Europe, and most permit cyclists of all skill levels, from recreational riders to elite competitors, to ride their tracks. Some anticipate that track racing's growing popularity will exceed its earlier successes.

Track bikes have a fixed rear cog that doesn't freewheel, and they don't have brakes. You will need a track bike if you are planning to compete, but many velodromes allow riders to use conventional road bikes. The tracks of a velodrome are oval, consisting of two 180-degree bends connected by two straight passages. They are usually composed of wood, concrete, or asphalt. They are steeply banked at angles ranging from 18 degrees to as much as 50 degrees. Tracks vary in length; the shorter the track, the steeper the banking. The pitch of the track allows riders to remain perpendicular to the surface while traveling at speed. The banking compensates for the way bicycles naturally lean into a turn, keeping them from being forced outward. The track is an exciting venue for training and racing.

Cyclists on the tracks don't shift gears; they maneuver their bikes, becoming extremely adept at handling in the process. In terms of competition, those who have ridden on a track have a huge advantage over cyclists who haven't. Track cycling sharpens your reactions, heightens your timing, improves and polishes

Eddie B's Track Workout

One of my favorite track workouts was developed by Edward Borysewicz, a famous American coach. Better known as "Eddie B," his cycling success at the 1984 Olympics in Los Angeles is legendary. Starting with a very long and slow warm-up behind a motorcycle, circle around the pole line (the innermost line on the velodrome surface). Riding at cruising speed, begin ramping up your intensity very gradually. Each rider in the group takes a turn riding behind the motorcycle, and after every lap or half lap, the lead rider pulls off toward the middle of the banking and then drifts to the back of the line. As the pace increases, the weaker riders drop off the back of the pack. For those that can hang with the group, the pace increases to more than 35 or 40 miles (56 or 64 km) per hour. At the end, only a few riders remain.

Next, riders do a series of six by three, or six laps ridden in groups of three people. The first three laps are motor-paced at a high rate of speed. In the last three laps, the lead rider passes the motorcycle and continues at full throttle for three more laps, changing the pace with each lap. Each interval has a new leader. Adjustments for cruise laps and equipment are made as needed. Next, riders do drills that are specific to the application. The pole is kept clear for the fastest session interval. Sprinters ride match-sprint drills both with and without motor pacing. Kilometer and pursuit specialists work on repeat starts, which is a fast start followed by a half lap at full speed. The final exercise consists of a few 4-by-200 (4 people over 200 meters) jumps that are performed very quickly to maximize leg response. Speed gradually diminishes during the cool-down period.

your sprinting, hones your intuitive instincts, and makes you think quickly on the fly. My best times and championship finishes have been produced after putting time in on the track.

Far more outdoor velodromes exist than indoor ones. If you do not have access to an indoor velodrome, consider doing some of your outdoor training on the track. The workouts are productive and fun, and you will not be disappointed.

POWER METERS

While you are training hard and seeing results, remember that masters cyclists must document the results of their workouts. Charting the physiological changes that occur with age allows you to work effectively around these issues with specific training methodologies. This practice also alerts you to your weaknesses and rewards you by showing your progress. Power meters help monitor your physiological changes and the corresponding changes in power output.

Power meters, or ergometers, have been on indoor-training bikes since the late 20th century. The industry has made many technological advances since their invention, especially in the last 10 years. These meters measure the cyclist's power output and provide essential information for defining and categorizing physiological thresholds, thus generating training results that are more quantifiable. You can use the data from training rides and races to illustrate and analyze training deficiencies and to catalog improvements.

Most power meters use strain gauges to measure the torque applied to the pedals and use the angular velocity of the wheel to calculate power (power = torque × angular velocity). This type of power meter is mounted on the bottom bracket, the crankset, or the free hub. Some of the newer power meters attach to the handlebars or stem and measure the opposing forces you encounter while cycling. Gravity, inertia, rolling resistance, wind resistance, and velocity combine to calculate your power output. Most power meters measure heart rate, speed, distance, and time, providing instant feedback on your physiological response. After your ride, you can download data to your computer and use your meter's software for in-depth analysis.

I use the CompuTrainer indoor system to look at every aspect of my clients' pedal strokes and to separate the curves for torque and power. The program generates a spreadsheet with values for wattage, heart rate, kilojoules, and the time elapsed for high, low, and average output. These accurately represent an athlete's efficiency. By downloading and tracking fitness changes, you can better understand the factors that limit your performance and begin the process of expanding them.

These physical and mental techniques will help you with your training, both indoors and out. Although their advantages and disadvantages are described in this chapter, each technique is only as good as the due diligence you offer. Successful workouts can be fun and rewarding, but they require dedication and discipline. There really is no such thing as a free lunch.

Training Zones

In *Training and Racing with a Power Meter,* Allen and Coggan present a power-output profile that charts performance for all levels of cyclists, from untrained amateurs to world-class athletes. These numbers are distressingly inappropriate for entry-level riders and masters. However, the authors do an excellent job of defining the categories of physical intensity. The progression of training takes many forms, and the process of measuring power output helps define zones based on physiological response. Target intensities for these zones are listed as percentages of functional threshold power (FTP), or the highest state of effort that a rider can maintain for an hour without fatigue. This value is roughly equivalent to lactate threshold; however, because a power meter measures power output, not levels of blood lactate, FTP is a measurable value that can be tracked.

If you have some training sessions completed using your power meter, you can estimate your FTP by downloading the data onto your computer and using the software that accompanied your unit. If you see a large dropoff in power output, this is a good indicator of your FTP. Check your manual for more information. If you are relying on a heart-rate monitor, you will need to determine what your maximum heart rate (MHR) is. There is a simple formula that you can use to estimate this value. If you are 30 years old or younger, simply subtract your age from 220. If you are older than thirty, use this formula to estimate MHR: MHR = 190-[(age-30)/2]. For example, if you are 50 years of age, your MHR = 190-[(50-30)/2]=180 beats per minute. The drawbacks of using a heart-rate monitor to gauge the intensity of your workouts is the tendency of the heart rate to drift higher during the workout even though the effort and intensity of the workout have not changed. This elevation in heart rate is usually due to dehydration and can be as much as 20 beats per minute during a 30-minute workout.

The following descriptions of training zones provide guidelines for the intensity of your workout.

Zone 1: Active Recovery

Fun rides with the family in which we smell the flowers and recover from hard training fall into the category of zone 1. Other examples include cool-down rides after a hard workout that break up the accumulated toxins in the soft tissue, or a spin class the day after a hard training ride. Recovery is essential for optimal progress, and the target intensity should be around 55 percent of FTP or about 50 to 60 percent of maximum heart rate.

Zone 2: Endurance

Workouts in zone 2 strengthen the heart muscles, increase the amount of cellular mitochondria, thus improving your body's capacity for repairing and rebuilding muscle tissue, and improve your ability to sustain energy. Unless you are unable to get outdoors at all, you probably will not do these workouts on your trainer. If you are housebound, a television or an interactive system will help you stay motivated. Training in zone 2 should last for two to three hours and should be punctuated with higher-intensity intervals and times to warm up and cool down. The target for workouts in zone 2 is 56 to 75 percent of FTP or 70 percent of maximum heart rate.

Zone 3: Tempo

Allen and Coggan call tempo workouts in zone 3 the meat and potatoes of training. This is the most productive training zone. However, in my coaching experience, cyclists and triathletes who spend too much time in this zone train themselves into a small box, becoming uncomfortable when they are forced to perform at a level that is more intense. The target for zone 3 is 76 to 90 percent of FTP or about 60 to 70 percent of maximum heart rate. You should be able to carry on a conversation at this level of exertion.

Zone 4: Sweet Spot

Allen and Coggan define zone 4 as the sweet spot of training, riding on the cusp between tempo and lactate threshold. This is an excellent training zone for building your FTP. Conditioning plays a big part in defining this level of intensity. Your target heart rate for this zone is 75 to 80 percent of maximum heart rate.

Zone 5: $\dot{V}O_2max$

Training in zone 5 will improve your $\dot{V}O_2max$, or the maximum volume of oxygen uptake. In racing, this kind of effort produces an attack with big wattage, and it is critical for breaking a race wide open and leaving the athletes who are not well trained gasping and reeling. VO_2max efforts are typically short, lasting between 15 seconds at the peak of an effort out of the saddle and three minutes. Zone 5 includes interval training with maximum effort between 106 and 120 percent of FTP or from 80 to 85 percent of maximum heart rate. Recovery periods should be performed in between, using the high intensity level of zone 2.

Zone 6: Anaerobic Capacity (AC)

If AC training had a color, it would be red. These timed intervals last a maximum of two minutes and are often much shorter. You cannot maintain this intensity aerobically since it requires more than 100 percent of your $\dot{V}O_2max$. These efforts push the pain meter solidly into the red zone! Training in zone 6 targets 121 to 150 percent of FTP or 85 to 95 percent of maximum heart rate.

Zone 7: Neuromuscular Power (NP)

Serious masters cyclists who want to complete the total power-based workout must participate in the ultimate on-bike explosion. Sprint intervals in big gears are NP-zone workouts. These efforts rarely last more than 10 or 15 seconds. You must have a high level of energy and good bike-handling skills to maintain control in extreme jumps while out of the saddle. In zone 7, you are working more than 150 percent of FTP or at greater than 95 percent of maximum heart rate.

Perfecting Bike-Handling Skills

When the weather and the roads are dry, it's time to take the bike outside and ride! Becoming a competent cyclist means acquiring the skill set and awareness of your surroundings needed for survival on the streets. In motor racing, drivers must attend and pass a driving course to enhance their skills before they can enter an open competition. Cycling has no such standards. In spite of the much higher speeds involved in auto racing, it is statistically far more dangerous to race a bicycle than a car. Anyone who has competed in or attended a higher-category criterium on a difficult cycling circuit will attest to the fact that many participants lack basic skills. One racer's mistake can result in a domino effect that brings down many riders, shredding their jerseys, leaving their flesh on the pavement, and mangling their bikes in the process.

America's first formal academy for teaching the art of cycling skills was the Dorset training group in Vermont, which was established by Wendy and Anne Cram in the early 1970s. The coaching agenda at Dorset, and at the school of champions in the early 1980s, involved the instruction of basic skills with classroom study and field sessions on the bike. To borrow a much-abused cliché, this is a proven methodology for teaching students techniques and skills that help them keep the rubber side down. Equipment has evolved, speeds have risen, and the rigors of competition have tightened, but no schools are currently

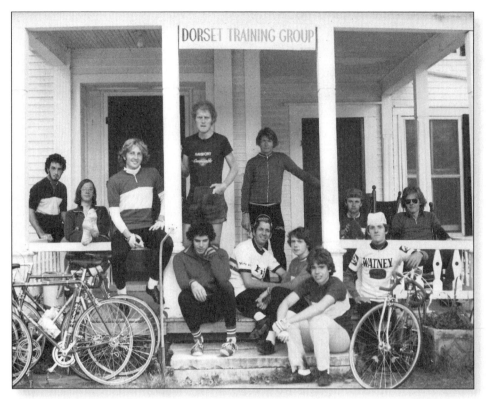

America's first organized training camp in Dorset, Vermont.

teaching these basic techniques to masters cyclists on an ongoing basis. There appears to be a notion among many cyclists that an activity they learned as children requires no further instruction. This *toy syndrome*, as I call it, continues to plague the sport of cycling.

The skills discussed in this chapter give cyclists more power, comfort, and safety for riding on the streets in traffic, negotiating turns and terrain, and dealing with road hazards, including other cyclists. Your goal should be to develop cycling skills that preserve life and limb and to gain bragging rights about medals, plaques, and trophies instead of about scar tissue and misaligned bones. Bike racing can become safer and more enjoyable when an adequate skill level is attained.

INDIVIDUAL RIDING SKILLS

Acquiring new cycling skills or improving those you already have is easier with professional instruction, but continual improvement comes with practice. Practicing new techniques will not only improve your skill level, but will also build your confidence and make you more comfortable negotiating roads that have ascents, descents, sharp turns, or other challenging features. Becoming a good climber requires patience, and when you have perfected your technical skills, you should schedule hill repeats in your training.

Climbing

Negotiating changing and challenging terrain is what cycling is all about. It can thrill, intimidate, frustrate, or delight. Unless you are a born-and-raised flat-lander, you are aware of the effects of gravity and the need to become a better, more-efficient climber. Maximizing your climbing potential requires improving your strength-to-weight ratio and technical skill. The steepness of the terrain and the length of the ascent will dictate when you remain seated and when it is necessary to rise out of the saddle.

Climbing in the Saddle

Honing your technique begins when you climb in the saddle and literally goes up from there. Imagine that you are climbing a hill with a grade between 2 and 3 percent. As you feel your rpm drop off, you shift into a smaller gear, increase your cadence, and maintain your speed. To keep your heart rate down, you try to stabilize your power by staying in the saddle, but the hill keeps getting steeper, and lactic acid begins to accumulate in your legs. Slide back in the saddle to leverage more force from your glutes and quadriceps. As the hill steepens further, try pointing your toes to bring the gastrocnemius and soleus (calf) muscles into firing position, boosting the back side of your stroke during hip flexion (see figure 6.1).

As the hill becomes steeper still, you must add more force to your hip flexors. Coach Ian Jackson refers to this scenario as the *coup de torchon*, which roughly translates to "the power of the dishtowel." Imagine holding a dishtowel tightly in both hands and then quickly moving your hands in circles. This image demonstrates the steady flow of power that should be distributed through the cranks as you pedal. To keep the center of the dishtowel in the same place, the pressure exerted by one hand must be equally exerted by the other in the opposite direction, then applied all the way around. Your objective is to connect the push of your pedal stroke with the pull to create a continuous application of power on the pedal for the entire stroke. Riding with a flat back and bent elbows lowers your center of gravity and engages the core muscles, delaying the accumulation of lactic acid in the primary muscles.

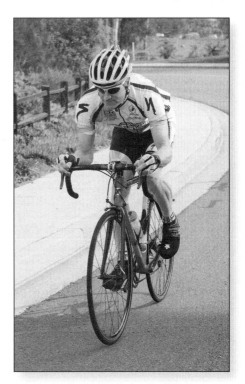

Figure 6.1 Climbing in the saddle.

As you climb, the hill becomes more precipitous, and you wonder if your tire is rubbing against the brake pad. At this point, many riders start losing ground. Their form deteriorates as they elevate their center of gravity, straighten their arms, and begin to fight the bike (see figure 6.2). Experienced masters cyclists remain low in the saddle, keeping their core muscles engaged and focusing on rhythmical and deep exhalations. Instead of yielding to the perceived forces of gravity, they dig a bit deeper while maintaining proper form. When your core muscles are effectively engaged, you enjoy greater stabilization, increased leverage, and a better distribution of muscular force and power. If the hill continues to challenge you and your rpm drops more than 10 percent below your target (for

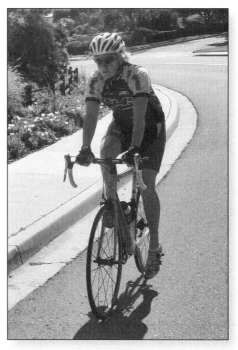

Figure 6.2 A less powerful, but more comfortable, recreational setup.

example, 65 to 70 rpm), it may be necessary to shift down, increase power, or leave the saddle. Climbing out of the saddle is usually the last resort since your rate of metabolic burn will climb as well.

The art of fast, efficient climbing requires the ability to recognize the precise moment when action is needed and to know what action to take. Should you shift down and stay seated, increase power output and risk being unable to sustain the effort, or leave the saddle and burn precious energy? At some point, it is prudent to climb out of the saddle since it produces more power and gives your muscles some much-needed relief. Delaying the decision too long will result in the loss of both speed and momentum. No magic formula exists for determining your course of action, but momentum must be preserved. Toggling between climbing in and out of the saddle may be a better choice for preserving power and for extending the life of your muscles.

Similarly, no magic formula exists for shifting while climbing. Your gear selection and shifting sequence depends on the available power, your fitness level, and the pitch of the climb. Cyclists who are more comfortable pushing big gears will climb using higher gears than those who like to spin the pedals at a higher rpm in lower gears. The length of the climb also dictates your approach. Shorter climbs allow you to produce more power than long climbs, in which conservation of energy is important. If you are starting to climb a long, gradual hill, use a gear that is comfortable and lets you maintain an rpm of about 90. When your cadence begins to slow down, downshift to an easier gear. If you are going to stand on the pedals, you may want to shift up to a higher gear so that you don't waste energy spinning.

Climbing out of the Saddle

As when climbing in the saddle, when you are out of the saddle during a climb, your goal is to maintain your heart rate and to increase forward momentum. Holding your hands on the brake hoods and your arms bent at the elbows and pointed slightly away from you, use your upper-body strength to leverage muscular force. To do this, pull on the handlebars while thrusting the leg on the same side. If done correctly, you will lighten the load on the major muscle groups in the lower body while improving the coordination of power and forward momentum. You may need to shift up with the extra power produced. The biomechanical requirements of climbing out of the saddle are very similar to those involved with sprinting. Sprinters apply an explosive burst of power to quickly bring the bike to maximum velocity, but climbing out of the saddle is a slower, more-sustained movement that brings you up the hill faster (see figure 6.3).

Gravity will win the battle if you surge on the pedals, pull and push your upper body forward or backward, or worse, pull your upper body up and down, disengaging the important core muscles. The primary force in moving the bicycle forward is generated at the 3 and 9 o'clock positions of the cranks. A common mistake among less-experienced riders is mistiming the thrust of the cranks. Power is dissipated at the top and bottom of the stroke, which is essentially a dead zone when out of the saddle. See figure 6.4 for an example of incorrect climbing out of the saddle by mistiming the thrust of the cranks.

Another common flaw is the tendency to rock the front wheel off center when climbing. Weaving up the road takes longer and costs you more energy, so try to maintain a smooth, circular pedal stroke. Balance your weight and center of gravity relative to the grade. If the grade is slight, you may remain seated or move out of the saddle to a position directly over the saddle and the crank axis. Steeper grades will require you to stand and position yourself forward to stay in front of the pedals (see figure 6.5).

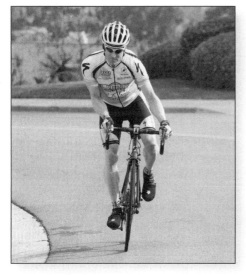

Figure 6.3 Climbing out of the saddle.

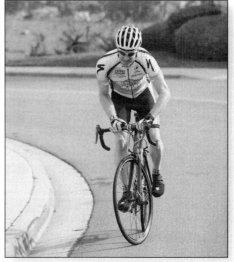

Figure 6.4 Incorrectly climbing out of the saddle.

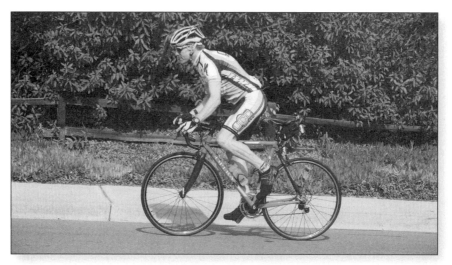

Figure 6.5 Climbing out of the saddle when the grade is steep.

Descending

You have worked hard to climb that hill, and now you are rewarded for your efforts with the thrill of a descent. Your center of gravity is low, you have moved back in the saddle, and your hands are in the drops as your speed begins to increase (see figure 6.6 for an example of correct and incorrect body positioning for descents). Safe, comfortable descents involve trusting your equipment and staying alert. Keep a sharp eye out for road hazards and wet or slick conditions. Anticipate the severity of each individual turn. Never bore into an unknown turn at high speed, and treat every descent with respect.

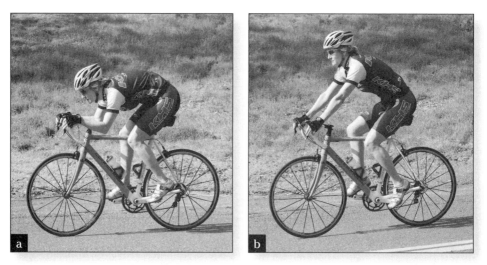

Figure 6.6 Body position when descending: *(a)* correct and *(b)* incorrect.

Practice on various grades, and learn the camber of the turns. Move your body around to get a feel for the position that gives you the best stability and aerodynamics. Level the cranks during descents to improve aerodynamics and balance and to accelerate at a faster rate. Sharper turns require that you adjust the cranks so that the inside crank is at the 12 o'clock position and the outside crank is at the 6 o'clock position. If you know of a descent with no traffic and want to experience the combination of descending and cornering, try running a short slalom down a hill. Use gentle maneuvers to sweep left and right, as if you were skiing down a mountain. This is one of the best training exercises for becoming comfortable descending at higher speeds. Be cautious and sensible, and always be mindful of traffic and road conditions.

In a group descent, you must exercise caution since other cyclists will be in close proximity and speeds can increase quickly. Anyone who has watched the Tour de France knows that even professional cyclists make mistakes. Crashes in group descents are most commonly caused by overlapping wheels. Hold your line, maintain a safe distance, and avoid nervous, squirrelly riders. You should also stay near the front of the pack since accidents occur more frequently in the back of large groups. Be alert and on the lookout for debris or irregularities in the pavement. Avoid making sudden moves and resist the urge to brake if you're gaining ground on the person in front of you. To slow your progress, simply sit up higher in the saddle to increase wind resistance.

Also note that if you are on a triathlon or time-trial bike with aero bars, be sure you're skilled enough to descend safely. A destabilizing, high-speed oscillation is more likely to happen with these bikes since the frame angles are steeper and the body is positioned forward. Don't panic! Gripping the top tube with your knees will immediately stop the oscillation and restore stability (see figure 6.7).

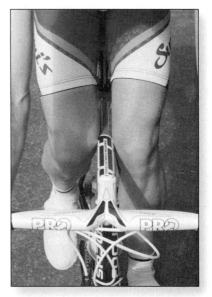

Figure 6.7 Technique for stabilizing the top tube.

Cornering

Experience is the most critical factor when it comes to cornering. Some years ago, I coached an international group of some of the era's best triathletes in the Tour of Redlands, an early-season professional stage race in southern California. The athletes were all powerful cycling time trialists, and I hoped those skills would make up for their universal lack of bike-racing skills, such as pack tactics and etiquette. In the tight circuit course of about a mile, riders were required to negotiate a series of sharp right and left turns in rapid succession.

Entering the turns in the thick of high-speed bike traffic was a challenge for seasoned pros since riders were positioned just inches from one another. The course demanded a high degree of bike-handling skill, and if they fell behind the peloton at 30 mph (48 kmph), they would never catch up.

From my position near the apex of one of the turns, I watched the pack bank from far edge to far edge, nearly clipping the apex where I was standing. I quickly jumped back and watched the riders exit wide and fast, losing a minimum of speed by using only a single gearshift. With my stopwatch, I timed my six triathletes. Three of them had some experience riding in a pack and positioned themselves in the group, staying there. The other three had problems in the turns. Lap after lap, the latter three lost ground in the turns, drifted off the back, then powered back to the pack on the straights. After 20 laps of this anaerobic seesaw, they were shelled off the back, where they were soon lapped and pulled from the race.

Cornering effectively is a technique that requires the ability to quickly judge the elements of a turn, which include sloping, curvature, traction, and other factors that limit speed. A bicycle, unlike an automobile, cannot be simply steered around a curve. Steering can bring the bike into a steeper bank than anticipated, and if you're going too fast, or if the road conditions aren't optimal, one or both wheels could lose traction and send you to the pavement. The bicycle must be leaned into the turn (see figure 6.8). You must estimate how much lean is needed to counteract the physical forces that want to project you and the bicycle in a straight line. The amount of lean depends on the speed traveled into the turn, the tightness of the turn, and the degree and direction of the road bank. When the road is sloped in the direction of the turn, less lean is needed, and the turn can be negotiated at faster speeds. However, if the road is sloped away from the turn, the lean angle will be greater, and slower speeds will be required through the turn. Keep your torso low and near to the top tube, and maintain weight on the outside pedal while easing up on the pressure to the inside pedal. You must also take care when negotiating roads that are wet or have potholes, loose gravel, and dirt.

Another technique for fast and efficient cornering is apexing, which is used to straighten out a turn. First, the turn is entered from the outer edge of the road to create the widest angle possible. Next, the apex, or midpoint of the turn, is cut on the inside. Finally, the turn is exited on the outside (see figure 6.9). Since the shortest distance between two points is a straight line, this technique shortens the dis-

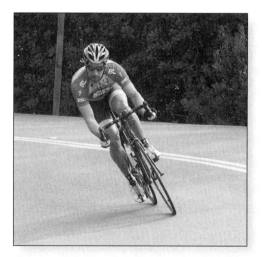

Figure 6.8 Leaning into the turn.

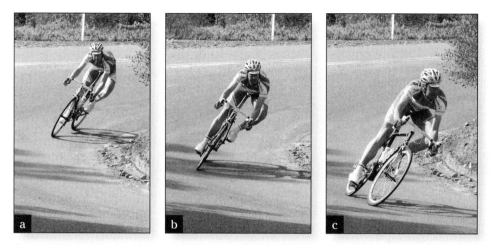

Figure 6.9 Apexing.

tance and lets you get through the turn with less lean and loss of speed. When approaching a curve, pick the line you want before entering the turn. The line you choose depends on the presence of automobile traffic and other cyclists. If you must brake in the turn, apply light, even pressure on both brake levers.

Certain techniques can be applied to maximize stability while cornering. With the inside crank at the 12 o'clock position, extend the knee into the turn while leaning your body into it (see figure 6.10*a*). Look through the corner without focusing on any particular object in your path. Inexperienced cyclists tend to watch their front wheels or look directly at objects, which can unintentionally carry them into the very objects they are trying to avoid. Additional stability can be gained by shifting your weight back in the saddle. Another trick is to apply pressure to the inside drop of the handlebar in the direction of the turn (see figure 6.10*b*). If your knee is already cocked out, and your momentum is

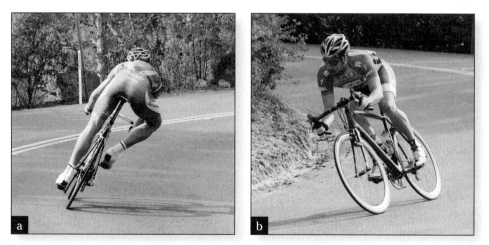

Figure 6.10 Maximize stability while cornering: *(a)* Extend the knee and body into the turn and *(b)* apply pressure to the inside drop of the handlebar in the direction of the turn.

increasing too rapidly, use your head and shoulder as an outrigger, leaning them into the direction of the turn. If you feel you are losing control, apply light, steady pressure to the brakes. If you spot gravel or other slippery debris, straighten your bike briefly as you pass through the area, resume your lean, and complete the turn. Above all, remain calm and respond to challenges with action rather than emotion.

Negotiating sharper turns at lower speeds or practicing in a parking lot with cones may help you to get a feel for the handling characteristics of your bike. Carving through a course of plastic cones or water bottles that are partially filled will do wonders to improve your cornering skills and build your confidence. This is a fun activity that few clubs practice. If you want to have some productive fun, invite some friends to do it with you. Bring a stopwatch.

Skillful cornering requires a lot of practice, and although helpful advice can be offered, these skills cannot be learned from a book. Relax and stay calm while cornering, especially during descents. When choosing your line through a turn, scan it for obstacles, potholes, and debris. Cornering reduces your speed, so you may want to either downshift before entering the turn or stay in the current gear and come out of the saddle, sprinting back up to speed as you exit. Avoid braking suddenly or making jerky movements, and maintain a smooth, fluid motion.

Regardless of your strength and speed, confidence comes from practicing, riding with experienced cyclists, and gradually building a sense of control and mastery. The best way to do this is by joining a bicycle club and regularly riding with a group. This environment usually teaches fledgling cyclists about riding etiquette: how and when to pass other cyclists, pointing out road hazards, signaling when stopping, and alerting cyclists behind you that a pedestrian is in the road or a car is pulling out. Effective communication among cyclists reduces the risk of accidents and injuries.

Off-Road Cornering

You should never negotiate single-track trails and fire roads with utter abandon, especially if you aren't familiar with them. Since four of my five broken bones from this sport have occurred in the dirt, I speak from experience. Off-road practice should progress in difficulty no matter how good a road cyclist you are. Many of the physical parameters of cornering on the road also apply off-road, but differences do exist. When riding through a downhill turn on a loose surface, try standing on the pedals in a crouched position instead of sliding back in the saddle. Bob Schultz, formerly a national NORBA champion in cross-country racing and a motocross racer, says, "Crouching forward on the pedals with your arms bent is an aggressive stance. The idea is to keep the upper body fluid and your elbows bent. Be ready to shift your weight backward or forward as needed."

Unlike cornering on the road, the crouched position helps absorb shock and allows you to make sharper turns faster by literally throwing your body weight into the turn. Instead of the traditional crank positions of 6 and 12 o'clock favored by road riders, Bob suggests adopting a pedal position of 3 and 9 o'clock for improved weight distribution and balance. Just as you would when executing a turn on gravel or soft dirt, always set your turn up wide and begin early enough to straighten slightly when you hit the loose spot. Cornering rapidly on a trail is very much like downhill skiing. Timing is critical. If you lose your rhythm on a fast set of turns, the error will be compounded as you go. The best downhillers seem to follow a policy of going in slowly and out fast; that is, they brake lightly before the turn, take the turn slowly, and power out of the turn. Ideally, you don't brake at all, but if you're coming in too fast, you do not want to wait until you're into the turn to brake.

Suspension systems on mountain bikes have changed the skill since they can corner safely with faster lines. However, even the best dual-suspension systems do little to prevent crashes if the speed of execution is beyond the skills of the rider. If you are competing off-road, arrive early and do a pre-run to scope out the terrain, establish your points for braking and shifting, and choose the correct line of entry and exit for the turns. Many top pros will run a particularly tough spot several times to try different lines before competition.

Cornering in Traffic

Cyclists must understand that automobile traffic is generally predictable because motorists usually have a straightforward agenda. Assume that motorists cannot see you and proceed with caution. Be especially cautious when you must cross several lanes of traffic to get to the left-turn lane, and signal your intention before crossing. Even when you signal, wait for a clearing in traffic before proceeding since not all drivers respect a cyclist's right to be on the road. Right turns are easy to negotiate, but try to exist harmoniously with motorists; never block a right lane when cars are turning right and you are not. Drivers are often uncomfortable turning in the presence of a cyclist. They will either sit impatiently behind you or speed up and turn in front of you, whether you're moving or not.

Braking

Two approaches to braking exist: One is used to stop the bike quickly to avoid a collision or other hazard, and the other consists of feathering the brakes to slow or stop forward progress. Feathering is the practice of applying light, even pressure on the front and rear brakes and is commonly used in most circumstances. There are times, however, when you may need to stop abruptly.

In my skills course, I frequently refer to emergency braking as a *hot stop*. The key to pulling off an effective stop is to remain calm. The technique I teach for stopping quickly is used only as an emergency maneuver to prevent a catastrophic accident. When a distracted motorist pulls out directly in front of you, or a stopped motorist swings a door open and obstructs the bike path, brakes should be a last resort. Allow yourself enough distance from parked

Cycling for Life

Victor Copeland

I worked with Vic when he was making the transition from triathlon to cycling in 1985. He has an impressive resumé with more than 50 national championship victories and at least one championship in each type of race contested on the road and the track. He has 12 gold medals from victories at the World Masters Games in Denmark, Australia, and Portland and holds 11 world track championships. "I've set at least 20 masters national track records and currently hold four world records, but I haven't approached 150 mph (242 kph) behind a race car," he says with a chuckle.

Vic still loves to compete and enjoys experimenting with different training programs. "My current goals are to not allow cycling to dominate my life too much and to include cross-training to enhance my overall fitness. I think easy running is great for recovery following hard, intense cycling sessions. It helps me keep my weight down and gives me another view of the world. It's also

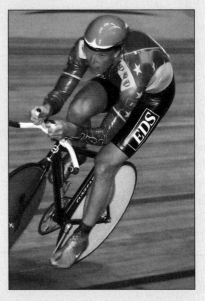

Dr. Vic Copeland, holder of numerous masters national and kilometer championship titles, on the track.

very good for preventing osteoporosis and keeping one's internal organs from sagging."

At the age of 67, Vic admits that he doesn't recover nearly as fast as he used to. "I try to compensate by training smarter. I do fewer high-intensity intervals, often skipping days, and do other sports activities for recovery. I work at drinking a lot of water and avoid alcohol, soft drinks, and sports drinks. I minimize carbs (particularly sugar) in my diet and eat mostly protein and good fats."

Two of Vic's four children are cyclists. His son, Zac, won the national sprint and kilometer championships and was responsible for getting his father into track racing. "I got tired of taking him to track practice and getting cold while I waited. So I got a track bike and started training with him." His youngest daughter, Joany, set the junior world kilometer record at the 1992 Olympic trials when she was 16, and she won the national criterium championship.

vehicles and ride at a reasonable speed so that you can easily maneuver around obstructions rather than applying your brakes. Another situation that may cause inexperienced cyclists to brake suddenly or to wobble is when a large vehicle passes in close proximity. The air displacement may cause a degree of buffeting when the turbulent air hits the cyclist. Do not panic! Grasp your handlebars firmly, hold your speed, and above all, hold your line.

When I was living in Staten Island, New York, my teammates and I in the U.S. Army would take the ferry to Battery Park and then ride up the Avenue of the Americas to Central Park to train. We were all national-team road and track racers. The trackies rode their fixed-gear bikes with no brakes, and we roadies maneuvered our safer, but more cumbersome, road bikes with brakes. The trackies inevitably beat us to the park by five minutes or more in the thick of Manhattan traffic. The moral of the story is that you can steer your way out of tight situations

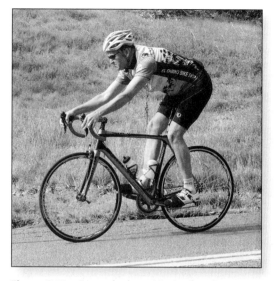

Figure 6.11 Correct body positioning for a hot stop.

more quickly than you can register and initiate a stop with brakes.

However, sometimes you have no choice but to brake. The hot stop is an important skill to understand and use in the event of an emergency. Suppose that the driver of an SUV spots a parking spot at the side of the road, abruptly tries to pull into it, and stops in your path. With substantial motor traffic on your left, you have nowhere to go. You only have a split second to identify the situation and respond, so the choice between maneuvering and braking must be instinctive and your reaction must be immediate. If you must stop, slip to the rear of the saddle to adjust your center of gravity (see figure 6.11). This action is accompanied by an approximate bias of two-thirds on the front brake and one-third on the rear brake. You will have very little time to slip back in the saddle and apply the front brakes. If your timing is off, you will find yourself going over the handlebars, especially if you're riding a steeply angled time-trial bike. When done properly, you can stop your bike in half the distance that it would normally take.

On roads that are wet, sandy, or strewn with debris, feathering the brakes is the only safe method of stopping. Braking in corners is usually a bad idea, especially when you are deep into a lean. If stopping is imperative, scrub off speed, applying equal pressure to the front and rear brakes to safely reduce speed.

Shifting

There is a science to shifting gears on a performance bicycle. As most cyclists know, gears make the job of traversing terrain easier. With 10-cog cassettes and triple-chain rings, the range of gears has increased to the point where gear spacing lets us use a single close-ratio cassette for nearly every type of riding we do. In the days when there were only five cogs on a screw-on steel cluster, it was necessary to change from one cluster to another during rides, depending on the pitch of climbs encountered. In the 1930s, before the derailleur was invented, riders used a hub with two cogs mounted on either side: a smaller one for the flats and a larger one for climbing. As they approached a hill, they dismounted, twisted off the rear wing nuts (quick-release hubs had not yet been invented), removed the wheel, turned it around, and refastened it to the bike for the climb. Of course, the entire procedure had to be repeated when they returned to flat roads. Modern gear spacing allows cyclists who are reasonably fit to climb almost any paved road.

Shifting a bicycle with the same technique you would use for a car with a manual transmission makes it easier for the engine (in this case, your body) to work. Maintaining a smooth speed with an efficient cadence keeps you from overtaxing your muscles and cardiorespiratory system. Measuring revolutions per minute is the standard method of determining the cadence of the drive train, which is made up of the cranks, pedals, chain, chain ring, and cogs. Whether you are a competitive or a recreational cyclist, your cadence needs to be as comfortable and smooth as possible, never jerky. Although training at a high cadence for prolonged periods can be valuable, it may not be the most efficient way to deliver power and speed. Some cyclists perform more efficiently pushing larger gears at a lower cadence. When you get the bike moving faster, shift gears and try to maintain cadence at the higher gear. If your legs are feeling the strain, it may be too late to shift up. When your body begins to rock and bob to find more power, it is definitely too late, and you have wasted an opportunity to capitalize on your momentum.

Shift one gear at a time, and avoid making big gear jumps between ranges. Modern bikes are indexed, and shifting is accompanied by an audible click. Before the shift index, shifters had to be eased from one gear to the next, turning as the cranks were turned to keep the chain operating smoothly. Shifting is now nearly foolproof. Do not try to downshift under pressure, such as when you wait too long to shift on a climb. Letting your revolutions per minute drop too low before shifting puts a great deal of stress on the drive train. Pedal lightly and smoothly, and avoid bogging down on the hills. When climbing a grade that is gradually steepening, shift before you start to struggle. This helps you maintain your cadence and time in the saddle. Listen to your bike and avoid crossing the chain over radical angles, such as the big chain ring and the larger cog in the rear. This will save wear and tear on your drive train and on your knees.

SKILLS FOR GROUP RIDING

Whether you call it a pack, a peloton, or a bunch, riding in a group allows you to cycle faster and conserve energy. It also teaches you to maneuver in close quarters. Group rides are a lot more fun than riding alone, and they will motivate you to ride harder than you would by yourself. Working the pack is a valuable skill that is mandatory for successful road racing. However, certain rules of the road must be observed to make riding in a pack a safe and enjoyable experience.

Pack Etiquette

Predictable behavior is critical when many people are riding in close proximity to one another. Unless you signal otherwise, other cyclists expect you to ride ahead at a constant speed and in a straight line. Remember to assume the speed of the person in front of you. Riders in a pack should use similar gears and cadence so that changes in speed and rates of acceleration are smoother. If you find yourself drifting up on the wheel in front of you too rapidly, sit up slightly, pedal softly, and let resistance from the wind slow you down. This strategy is much better than braking, which may cause panic or a chain reaction in the pack. On the other hand, if the person in front of you steps up the pace and creates a gap, avoid sudden acceleration. Pick up the pace slowly to conserve energy. Avoid opening a large gap between yourself and the person behind you.

You should also assume an aerodynamic position when you are left exposed in the wind. Stay out of your aero bars in a group! When you are in your aero bars, you do not have ready access to your brakes. In close quarters, these bars are more likely to be the cause of a crash, to say nothing of the likelihood for greater injury. The lead riders in a group are responsible for providing visual feedback to the other cyclists. Issue a verbal warning for potholes and road kill, and point out pedestrians or small obstacles with your finger.

If you aren't making an effort to advance in a pack, then you are probably losing ground to riders who are. My approach to pack riding is to advance, then drift back only far enough to remain with the people who are dictating the race pace. Avoid slipping too far to the rear since you are more likely to be dropped as soon as a gap opens up. More crashes occur at the back, largely due to the whiplash effect from problems farther up the line. The middle of the pack is safer and more protected. Sit in the first third of the field. If you sit too close to the front, you will waste energy trying to stay in the rotation of a pace line. On the other hand, experienced riders who sit just behind the leaders are close enough to strike if the going gets tough, or to respond to the threat of a breakaway.

While riding in a pack, you will inevitably experience the echelon, an advanced technique that requires practice in a group. Echelons, as shown in figure 6.12, form when crosswinds are present. The sweet spot, or the location with the least wind resistance, is no longer behind the rider in front. Instead, the sweet spot lies to one side or the other, depending on the direction of the wind. Riders extend a simple line formation into a unit of protection against crosswinds that is more complete. They always pull into the wind, and each person in the formation moves over one slot as the leader pulls off. The leader drops off directly behind the line of riders to gain maximum protection. Never allow your wheels to overlap with another cyclist's. This is the primary cause of group crashes.

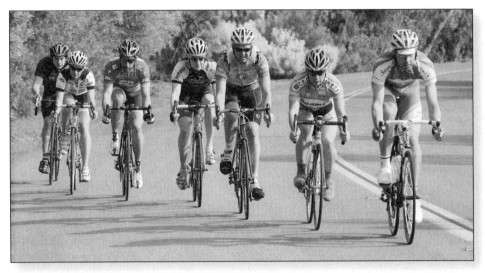

Figure 6.12 An echelon.

Looking Ahead and Behind

One of the first things I learned about riding in a pack was to keep my eyes trained ahead at all times. If you become mesmerized, watching the rear hub of the bike in front of you, you may not see the car pull out of a side street a hundred yards (91 m) in front of the leaders. Scan the road ahead and watch the bodies of the next few riders in front of you. Learn to identify and avoid nervous and inexperienced riders; they grip the bars tightly, brake frequently, and allow their front wheels to wobble periodically, making them treacherous in close quarters. Watch out for road hazards, sudden turns, blind intersections, and inattentive motorists. Assume that motorists do not see you and act accordingly since you most likely will lose in a confrontation with an automobile. Motorists are worried about other motorists, and cyclists are a secondary concern. You must take responsibility for your own safety.

Novice cyclists tend to ride with a stiff upper body, which puts the torso under continuous stress and makes looking behind more difficult. Looking over your shoulder can turn the bars as well, causing your bike to veer into a curb, another cyclist, or out into traffic. To avoid swerving, relax your upper body and bend your elbows. Practice redistributing your weight as you turn and see how close you can stay to a lane line. After your balance and control improve, try the exercise in traffic. You can improve your range of motion to easily look over your shoulder with gentle, prolonged (hold for six deep breaths) spinal twists in both directions.

Some cyclists like to attach rearview mirrors to their helmets or handlebars. They can be useful for commuting by bicycle through congested city streets; however, I don't recommend them for group rides. You need to be aware of the cyclists around you in a pack and your physical surroundings so that you can

Pace Lines

When you have two or more riders, with five or six being ideal, you can build a pace line (see figure 6.13). A pace line is nothing more than a formally defined segment of the pack that has a specific agenda, such as chasing a breakaway group or participating in a break. In other words, it is a strategy for working together to go faster while preserving energy. Even at 15 mph (24 kph), the drafting provided by a pace line can be effective since beyond that speed, your effort increasingly goes toward overcoming wind resistance. Serious, experienced riders will maintain a space of 12 to 24 inches (30-60 cm) between bikes; beginners are more comfortable with a gap between 24 and 36 inches (90 cm). Avoid overlapping wheels, and observe the same etiquette practices as for riding in a pack.

Ideally, a pace line's mechanics should mesh like the gears on a fine Swiss watch. When a rider takes a pull at the front, the effort should be shorter when you're feeling weak, longer when you're feeling strong, and always long enough to let the previous leader drop to the back. When you drop to the back, glance over your shoulder to watch for overtaking traffic, signal with a wave of your palm or a shake of your elbow, pull off toward the line of traffic, and then immediately soft pedal until the group is past. When the front wheel of the last rider in the line emerges in your peripheral vision, start picking up the pace and blend smoothly into the back of the line. Don't make the mistake of pulling out of the pace line and moving 5 feet (1.5 m) away. This can be dangerous in traffic and quite taxing since you have greater exposure to the wind. Keep a tight line when returning to the back of the pack, no more than one-and-a-half bike widths away from the others. When I was a member of the national team and rode the 100K team time trial in the Olympic, World, and Pan American Games, I remember being so close to my teammates that we would brush elbows on the return. This situation is not advisable, but it does illustrate how a tight and efficient pace line can work.

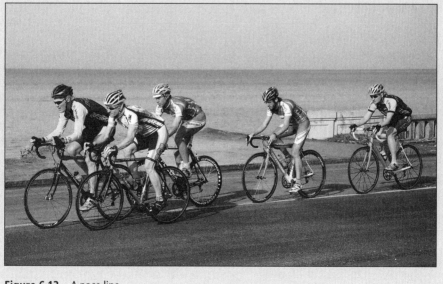

Figure 6.13 A pace line.

react appropriately. Develop your instincts, using all of your senses to detect approaching vehicles and identify hazards. Never use headphones or earbuds while riding a bicycle. This practice essentially deafens you. You cannot hear motor vehicles or cyclists approaching from the rear or verbal warnings from others.

Climbing in a Pack

The first lesson for climbing in a pack is to maintain a comfortable tempo. Begin a long, gradual climb in your comfort zone. For most people, this means an rpm of 90. If your cadence starts to slip, slightly reduce the pressure on the pedals and shift down to an easier gear. On longer climbs, you should be at the front. If you have to downshift, you may slide back, but you won't fall off the back of the pack. If you slack off for even a second to jump when out of the saddle, the loss of momentum will drop you back into the wheel directly behind you. This is a potentially dangerous move since it can cause an immediate overlap of wheels that may take down the person behind you. Instead, try to maintain your cadence and apply constant pressure on the pedals. This may require you to shift into a higher gear. Since cadence and speed can be difficult to maintain during a climb, you usually see the pack spread out.

Climbing separates riders by their ratios of strength to weight. If you want to hang with the leaders, you must improve your personal strength-to-weight numbers by doing hill repeats of varying lengths, and perhaps by reducing your weight. If you don't think weighing a few extra pounds is significant, pick up a 5- or 10-pound (2 to 4.5 kg) dumbbell and imagine hauling it up a steep hill. When climbing, try to keep your shoulders loose and relaxed. Breathe deeply and rhythmically, engage your core muscles, and stay low in the saddle with your elbows bent.

Descending in a Pack

Flying down a hill with a bunch of other cyclists can be a bit intimidating if you aren't experienced. If someone goes down, others are likely to pile on top. At high speeds, a lot of flesh can be left on the pavement. Typically, unless you're a professional, the pack spreads out a bit so that the cyclists have more space between them. Do not center on the wheel in front of you. Instead, keep your front wheel behind and off to the side of the rear wheel of the cyclist ahead of you. The cyclists behind you are depending on you for a safe descent. Make no unexpected moves, avoid braking, and stay alert.

Cornering in a Pack

The basic principles of cornering that were previously discussed hold true in a group as well. The best strategy for cornering with other cyclists can be summed up in three words: Hold your line. Nothing is more frightening and disconcerting than a rider who does not respect this rule and changes lines in the middle of a turn, causing the other cyclists to brake or change their lines. This is extremely dangerous since it may lead to a chain-reaction collision that causes many in the group to go down. Much grief can be prevented by identifying squirrelly cyclists and avoiding them. Assume the speed of the cyclists in the turn ahead of you, pedal when they do, and maintain the gaps between riders.

Don't expect to master all of these techniques in a brief period. It takes years of training and racing with all kinds of cyclists to become a master. To become comfortable riding in close quarters, bite off a little at a time and integrate it into your training routine until it becomes second nature. Be aware that two general types of turning maneuvers exist: those that are steered and those that are not. Save your skin by practicing both types of maneuvers with pylons, as previously described. Start slowly and build your technique. As with skiing, speed comes with experience. Remember, there is a huge difference between simply taking risks and carefully calculating them.

Planning a Performance Diet

Since you literally are what you eat, nutrition is one of the most important considerations for masters athletes. The foods and supplements that make up your diet support your health, energy level, and ability to recovery from exercise. Masters athletes who train 12 to 14 hours each week need a different level of nutrition than those who only ride on the weekends. This chapter presents the array of nutritional choices available and discusses which nutrients you need and why.

We get most of our nutrients from food, so our discussion begins with the pyramid outlined by the U.S. Department of Agriculture (USDA). You will learn which foods satisfy your hunger while supplying your body with ample nutrients. Your need for the macronutrients (carbohydrate, protein, fat, and water) in food depends on your level of activity. Athletes who engage in high levels of training and competition burn calories at higher rates, so along with an increased food intake, they may need to supplement their diet with a spectrum of micronutrients (vitamins and minerals). Masters cyclists metabolize food at about the same rate that their younger counterparts do, but they have a host of other nutritional concerns that warrant consideration, including calcium deficiencies. Regardless of their age, endurance athletes should be concerned with the accumulation of free radicals in the body. High levels of free radicals cause cellular damage that can seriously compromise health and recovery after activities. However, these levels can be greatly reduced by eating foods containing antioxidants and perhaps taking antioxidant supplements. Food should be your primary source for these compounds, but if you decide you need to take supplements, exercise restraint, as an excess of antioxidants in the system can become pro-oxidative.

THE NUTRITION PYRAMID

The nutrition pyramid outlined by the USDA consists of the following food groups: grains, vegetables, fruits, dairy products, meat and beans (meat, poultry, fish, dried beans, eggs, and nuts), oils, and descretionary calories (see figure 7.1). The grain group is divided into whole grains and refined grains. Fruits include fruit juices. Vegetables are classified as dark green, orange, starchy, or other, which consists of all other vegetables and vegetable juices. Oils are fats that are monounsaturated or polyunsaturated (liquid at room temperature). The guidelines for intake from this group recommend fats from fish, nuts, and vegetables. However, you should limit your intake of solid (saturated) fats, such as butter, stick margarine, shortening, and lard, which are listed among "discretionary calories." Another facet of the pyramid is labeled physical activity, which is divided into moderate and vigorous exercises. Examples are provided

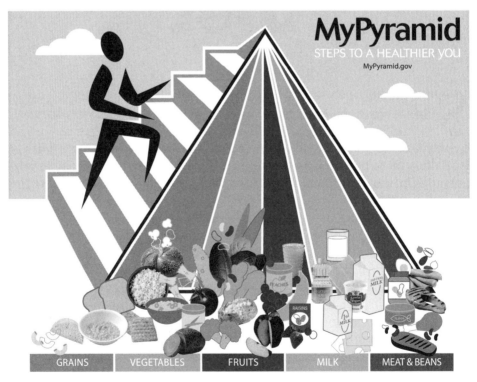

Figure 7.1 The food pyramid.

U.S. Department of Agriculture

for each category. The model stresses a balance between diet and physical activity and suggests that we engage in at least 30 minutes of moderate physical activity each day.

The dietary guidelines emphasize consuming vegetables, fruits, whole grains, and dairy products that are either nonfat or low in fat. Other recommended foods are lean meats, poultry, fish, beans, eggs, nuts, and small amounts of saturated fat, trans fat, salt (sodium), and sugar. Keep in mind that these recommendations are for the general public aged 2 and older. They do not take dietary restrictions, health issues, or special needs into account. Masters athletes have special needs since they place a much greater physical demand on their bodies than average people do. Caloric requirements differ from athlete to athlete based on genetics, metabolic rate, build, and degree of physical activity. Masters athletes should make some general modifications to the pyramid for a more efficient and healthful diet.

Grains

Grains, such as oats, wheat, rice, and barley, have been historically important for human survival. People have been eating whole grains for thousands of years and may have cultivated them as far back as 9000 BC in the part of the Middle East that was known as the Fertile Crescent. When kept dry and free of pests, grains could be stored for long periods to be used during winter months or in times of famine.

Efficient methods of processing have been developed in which the natural bran (fiber) and the germ are removed from the grains used for white bread, pasta, and white rice. Although five vitamins and minerals are added to the grains again after processing, many naturally occurring antioxidants, vitamins, minerals, and fiber are removed and not replaced. Although refined grains are indeed complex carbohydrates, the body tends to metabolize them more quickly than whole grains. Whole grains provide a variety of important vitamins, minerals, phytonutrients, and fiber that will give you more sustained energy for riding.

Whole grains have protein and certain phytonutrients that are usually absent from fruits and vegetables. They are a rich source of saponins, contain vitamin E, and some contain phytoestrogens. Phytoestrogens, which are nonsteroidal plant compounds that closely mimic estrogen, include lignans, flavonoids, and coumestans. Some studies on phytoestrogens suggest that they reduce breast and prostate cancers and cardiovascular disease, protect against osteoporosis, and provide relief from menopausal symptoms. Flax seed and soybeans, which are classified under seeds and legumes, respectively, are by far the foods richest in phytoestrogens.

Vegetables

Vegetables are veritable treasure troves of nutrients that benefit the human body, especially when eaten raw. They are full of vitamins, fiber, minerals, and antioxidants. Cyclists must include them in their diet if they want to maximize their performance. Available in every color of the rainbow, vegetables are rich in phytonutrients that offer a wide array of benefits, including anti-inflammatory and anticancer properties. During physical activity, cyclists generate free radicals that damage muscle tissue through oxidation. Vegetables contain antioxidants that neutralize free radicals and help repair cellular damage.

Phytonutrients are compounds that naturally occur in plants, such as beta-carotene, lycopene, and sulforaphane. They are the biologically active components of pigments in the skin of fruits and vegetables, and they are responsible for the color, scent, and flavor. The health benefits of phytonutrients include antioxidant protection from free radicals, heart health, and improved vision. For example, lycopene is the phytonutrient that gives tomatoes their color. It is a strong antioxidant and has been shown to reduce the risk of heart disease.

Let's consider some vegetables and their features. An artichoke (120 grams) contains vitamin C, magnesium, folate, potassium, and 10 grams of fiber. One-half cup of lentils has 8 grams of fiber and many healthy compounds, including saponins, a class of phytonutrients that may lower cholesterol and blood-glucose levels. One cup of broccoli has 6 grams of fiber and hefty quantities of vitamins and minerals. It also has sulforaphane, a phytonutrient that, according to a study conducted at Rutgers University and published online in *Carcinogenesis*, has significant anticancer effects.

Green vegetables, such as broccoli, contain phytochemicals that aid digestion. Leafy greens, such as spinach, kale, and collard greens, help keep your eyes healthy. Some green vegetables are high in beta-carotene. Beta-carotene is a powerful antioxidant that is converted to vitamin A and promotes good vision and a healthy immune system. Several green vegetables are rich in potassium, which helps your muscles, including your heart, fire correctly. They also contain calcium for healthy bones. Greens that belong to the cabbage family offer anticancer phytonutrients. Asparagus is rich in carotenoids, lutein, vitamin A, folate, iron, and more. The color of red and yellow vegetables, such as carrots, yams, and yellow peppers, comes from carotenoids. Carotenoids are metabolized into nutrients like vitamin A, which promotes iron absorption in people who are anemic. Tomatoes contain lycopene, which is thought to offer protection from ultraviolet rays that can damage to the skin.

If you prefer your vegetables cooked, use restraint since the level of water soluble nutrients tends to decline the more they are cooked. Lightly steam them until they are tender but still crisp. Add raw vegetables to your salads, or prepare raw-vegetable soups in your blender with herbs, onion, garlic, lemon juice, salt, and pepper for added flavor.

If you avoid onions because you think they cause breath odor, you may want to rethink that choice. Onions contain vitamins B_6 and C, chromium, biotin, and fiber. They also contain folic acid, vitamin B_1, potassium, flavonoids (antioxidants), phenolic acids (antioxidants), sterols, and saponins. Plant sterols help reduce blood cholesterol and keep the blood vessels healthy and flexible.

Onions and their extracts reduce the amount of lipids (fats) in the blood, prevent the formation of clots, and decrease blood pressure. They have also been found to significantly lower blood glucose. Garlic produces similar effects. If you have not been eating onions and garlic, consider adding them to your diet for their wonderful health benefits.

Fruits

Fruits are another rich source of vitamins, minerals, and phytonutrients. Since they are usually eaten raw, you can enjoy their full nutritional value. Fruits come in all shapes, sizes, and colors. Like vegetables, they contain plant sterols. They have little or no protein and fat with the exception of avocados and coconuts, and are essentially carbohydrate: complex nonstarch polysaccharides (fiber), sugars, and water.

Citrus fruits are generally thought of as a rich source of vitamin C, but they are also an excellent source of fiber, potassium, folate, and thiamin, and they also contain calcium, niacin, vitamin B_6, phosphorus, magnesium, and copper. They also provide health benefits in terms of phytonutrients and aromatherapy. Many other fruits also provide health benefits. Dr. Bill Sears, who is a long-time pediatrician concerned with family nutrition, a masters endurance cyclist, and a triathlete, lists his top 10 fruits based on their content of vitamin C, fiber, carotenoids, calcium, and folic acid. He ranks avocados in the number 1 slot, followed by papayas, guavas, cantaloupe, dried apricots, mangoes, strawberries, kiwi fruit, and grapefruit.

Bananas have always been popular with cyclists as an energy booster. They have virtually no saturated fat or sodium, and they're a good source of dietary fiber, vitamins C and B_6, potassium, and magnesium. They have a high glycemic index (GI) of 89. Foods with high glycemic indexes will give a cyclist a quick boost of energy during a ride but do not offer sustainable energy.

The glycemic index was conceptualized by Dr. David Jenkins and his colleagues at the University of Toronto in the early 1980s. It measures the effects of carbohydrate on the level of glucose in the blood: carbohydrate that breaks down quickly, releasing sugar into the bloodstream, has high indexes. Those types that break down more slowly have lower indices. Glucose is used as the reference food with a glycemic index of 100. On the Internet you can easily find tables of foods with their corresponding glycemic indexes.

Berries are excellent sources of vitamins and phytonutrients and have the highest antioxidant level of all fruits. All berries are rich in vitamin C. For example, one cup of strawberries contains 100 mg of vitamin C, which is slightly less than what is found in a cup of orange juice. A cup of strawberries also contains small amounts of calcium, magnesium, folate, and potassium, and it's only 53 calories. Cranberries and blueberries contain tannins (plant polyphenols) that prevent E. coli bacteria, the most common cause of urinary tract infections, from adhering to the walls of the bladder and causing an infection. They also contain

Facts About Fiber

Dietary fiber, or roughage, is a key component of fruits and vegetables that plays an important role. The primary function of the colon is to complete the digestion process by removing excess water from waste material. If waste passes through the colon too rapidly, too much water will remain, causing loose bowels or diarrhea. If waste passes too slowly, hard bowel movements, constipation, or hemorrhoids may occur. Fiber, such as cellulose, pectins, gums, mucilages, and lignans, forms the structure of the plant and isn't digestible. It facilitates the passage of waste through the colon by expanding the colon walls and increasing the wavelike contractions that move the material toward excretion. Soluble fibers bind to fatty materials in the intestines so they can be eliminated, thus reducing the level of low-density lipoprotein (bad cholesterol) in the body.

Fiber also slows the rate at which fruits and vegetables are metabolized, thereby affecting the glycemic index of the food. Starchy vegetables, such as sweet corn, and potatoes, are relatively low in fiber and have high glycemic indices. How you cook a vegetable can affect the GI. For example, white potatoes, when steamed, mashed, boiled, fried, microwaved, or baked, have glycemic indices of 83, 93, 100, 104, 107, 117, and 158, respectively. Consider eating yams or sweet potatoes, which have much more fiber and glycemic indexes of 63 and 73, respectively. As different foods are often consumed at the same time, their glycemic indexes will be affected by what is eaten with them.

Avocados have 11 to 16 grams of fiber, depending on the size and variety, and a negligible GI. They are rich in vitamins, minerals, and lutein, a phytonutrient. Other healthy choices that are high in fiber are lentils, broccoli, and artichokes.

phytonutrients: beta-carotene, zeaxanthin, and lutein. Zeaxanthin and lutein are structurally similar and are found in the macula of the retina. They have been found to protect against cataract development and age-related macular degeneration, which results in loss of vision. A berry that has been getting a lot of attention recently is the acai berry, which comes from the acai palms in the rainforests of Central and South America. It is a good source of anthocyanins, flavonoids (antioxidants), fiber, and omega fat.

Milk

Milk and dairy products are excellent sources of protein, calcium, potassium, and vitamin A. Milk is often fortified with vitamin D. Yogurt is a cultured milk product, which is produced by adding probiotics (good bacteria similar to those that exist naturally in human intestines) to milk or cream, yielding food that is thick, creamy, and rich in nutrients. Yogurt helps maintain a healthy digestive system, and one cup has as much potassium as a banana. Depending on the type, cheese is also a rich source of protein, phosphorus, vitamin A, and folate. If you have difficulty digesting dairy, try cheddar and Swiss cheeses, which have little lactose.

Meat and Beans

The meat and bean group covers a lot of territory and includes all types of meat (beef, lamb, pork), eggs, shellfish, nuts, seeds, and poultry, all rich sources of protein. Proteins are structurally complex polymers that make up about 50 percent of the dry weight of cells. A polymer is a chain of simple repeating units. In the case of protein, these repeating units are amino acids. We eat protein for the essential amino acids.

Eggs have gotten a bad rap over the years but are extremely good sources of protein. Although one egg does have 213 milligrams of cholesterol, dietary cholesterol affects some individuals more than others, and earlier studies may have over-exaggerated the negative impact of eggs for most people. They raise the levels of both high-density lipoprotein (HDL) and low-density lipoprotein (LDL), so the ratio of HDL to LDL cholesterol remains the same. Eggs are very nutritious with 72 calories, 6 grams of protein, and only 2 grams of saturated fat. They also contain vitamins E and B_{12}, riboflavin, folic acid, calcium, zinc, iron, and essential fatty acids.

All varieties of fish, including shellfish, are also on the list of good types of protein. Although the leanest grades of beef have also been included, avoid prime rib, ribeyes, T-bones, and other cuts that are marbled with fat. Since these cuts are also the most expensive, you'll ease the pressure on your wallet by choosing loin, round, sirloin, and top round cuts instead. The list of approved meats also includes pork tenderloins and loin roasts, and skinless chicken and turkey breasts, which are low in cholesterol and fat. Beans, split peas, and lentils, which have low glycemic indexes, provide all of the essential amino acids when eaten with grains. Small amounts of lean meats already have all of the essential amino acids.

Milk, cheeses, and yogurts with fat contents of zero and one-percent are good, but beware of flavored yogurts that are full of sugar. Instead, top unflavored, unsweetened yogurt with fresh fruit or nuts. Full-fat dairy products contain cholesterol and are high in saturated fat. Their benefits come from the calcium, vitamin A, protein, and phosphorus present, not the fat, so choose the low-fat varieties.

Oils

Oils are mostly made of unsaturated fat that are liquid at room temperature. Vegetable oil is usually a blend of soybean, corn, sunflower, and palm oils. It contains both saturated and unsaturated fats and may contain undesirable trans fat. Canola oil has a very low level of saturated fat and a high level of monounsaturated fat and linolenic acid. Olive oil is also low in saturated fat and high in monounsaturated fats and linoleic acid. Monounsaturated oils promote a healthy ratio of HDL and LDL (good and bad cholesterols). Linoleic acid, an omega-6 fatty acid, and linolenic acid, an omega-3 fatty acid, are essential fatty acids (EFA). The body does not manufacture them, so they must be obtained from the diet, and they are vital for proper function of the cardiorespiratory, musculoskeletal, gastrointestinal, and immune systems.

Discretionary Calories

Let's say you are budgeting a specific number of calories to be consumed each day. You have line items for foods that you must eat to keep your body well nourished and healthy. Any leftover calories are considered extra or discretionary and should usually be limited to fewer than 300 per day. This category includes sugary foods, saturated fat, and alcoholic beverages. The more calories you burn during training, the more discretionary calories you may consume without negative effects.

MACRONUTRIENTS AND MICRONUTRIENTS

All nutrients can be broken down into two categories: essential and nonessential. Nonessential nutrients can be synthesized by the body, but essential nutrients must be obtained from food or through supplementation. Nutrition begins with the consumption of foods. The process of digestion commences in the mouth when food meets enzymes in the saliva and then continues as food moves through the gastrointestinal tract.

During digestion, macro- and micronutrients are absorbed into the bloodstream through the lining of the small intestine and are carried to every part of the body. When they reach the cells, these products are either used to make the carbohydrate, protein, and fat in human tissue, or are metabolized for energy. Glucose that is not quickly used is converted into glycogen (long, branched chains of glucose) in the liver and muscles before being stored. The adage about computers, "garbage in, garbage out," can be applied to the human body. If you eat garbage, your athletic performance and recovery will suffer.

Macronutrients

Macronutrients make up the majority of a person's diet and include protein, carbohydrate, fat, macrominerals, and water. These substances are required in large amounts for growth and maintenance of the body. Macronutrients supply energy in the form of calories; there are 4 calories for every gram of protein, 4 calories per gram of carbohydrate, and 9 calories per gram of fat.

Carbohydrate

Carbohydrate is an organic compound that contains carbon, hydrogen, and oxygen. It is basically a hydrate of carbon. A carbohydrate is also known as a *saccharide*, a natural carbohydrate that plays a major role in biological processes. Carbohydrates can be divided into three categories: simple carbohydrates, complex carbohydrates, and fiber.

Consuming Soft Drinks and Alcohol

While soft drinks contribute calories and carbohydrate, they provide no other vitamins, minerals, or phytochemicals. These beverages are often referred to as "empty calories" because of the absence of any nutritional value. Alcohol also provides calories, but they are burned in a way that is somewhat different from other calories. Some alcoholic beverages contain beneficial phytochemicals, but excessive consumption can be harmful to your health and your athletic performance.

Soft Drinks

Many sodas, especially colas, contain phosphoric acid to preserve and sharpen the flavor. Phosphoric acid is known to cause bone loss in people who do not get enough calcium in their diet since it extracts calcium from the bones, increasing your risk for osteopenia or osteoporosis. The sugar content of most regular sodas is between 7 and 14 percent, including sucrose, fructose, and glucose. A 12-ounce (350 ml) can of cola has 140 calories, which all come all from sugar.

Wine

Wine is rich in flavonoids, vitamin B, and potassium. It facilitates the production of gastric juices, aiding digestion. It also contains antioxidants, such as a phytoestrogen called resveratrol that has been shown to slow the formation and growth of cancers. Much ado has been made in recent years over the benefits of drinking wine, especially red wine. Although many benefits exist, be aware that these reports refer to moderate consumption, which is defined by the American Heart Association as one or two 4-ounce (120 ml) glasses per day. Although wine offers benefits in moderate amounts, the consumption of excessive amounts has a negative effect on life expectancy. It can cause cancer, especially breast cancer in women. Alcohol also has many calories, and it stimulates the appetite, which can lead to obesity and related health issues when consumed in excess.

Beer

One 12-ounce (350 ml) serving of regular beer has 153 calories, 2 grams of protein, 14 milligrams of calcium, 21 milligrams of magnesium, 50 grams of phosphorus, 96 milligrams of potassium, 14 milligrams of sodium, a trace of zinc, and 1 milligram of thiamin. Consuming three beers means taking in a whopping 459 calories! Even two beers per day over a week's time accumulates to more than 2,000 calories per week.

Like wine, beer promotes a healthier ratio of HDL to LDL. A liter of beer contains between 10 and 45 percent of the recommended daily dose of folate, which may help decrease the level of homocysteine in the blood, minimizing the risk of cardiovascular disease. According to *The Food Paper* and a number of other sources, the hops in beer contain plant sterols with antioxidant properties similar to those in wine, which may offer protection against cancer. Recent studies indicate that beer, like red wine, improves arterial elasticity, reducing risk for hypertension, stroke, and heart disease. However, women are advised to have no more than one beer per day, and men should limit their intake to two beers.

Simple Carbohydrates Simple carbohydrates consist of monosaccharides and disaccharides. Table sugar, or cane sugar, is made of sucrose, a disaccharide that is composed of glucose and fructose. It is commonly added to cereals, hot beverages, lemonade, tea, baked beans, and baked goods, such as cakes, pies, and cookies. It can be found in ketchup, sweet pickles, jams and jellies, syrups, candies, and ice cream. The average American consumes 152 pounds (70 kg) of sugar each year, which amounts to an alarming 3 pounds (1.4 kg) each week! Sugar is cheap, tasty, and habit-forming. Food-processing companies, including fast-food restaurants, add liberal amounts to their products.

Some people are more sensitive to fluctuations in blood sugar levels than others, feeling energized at first and then fatigued. Fifty percent of table sugar is glucose, which enters the bloodstream quickly, causing an increase in blood sugar. This signals the pancreas to send insulin into the bloodstream to move the glucose into muscle cells for energy. When blood sugar levels fluctuate significantly, the impact on energy level may be felt by people who are sensitive to these changes. Sugars, such as those in soft drinks and sweets, are providing calories without any nutritional benefits. All excess calories that are not burned by exercise and daily activities will be stored as fat, including the calories that come from sugar.

Fruits contain glucose, sucrose, and fructose. These types of sugar present the same issues as cane sugar when imbibed in the form of juices or when added to processed foods. Fructose is added in large quantities to soft drinks in the form of high-fructose corn syrup (HFCS). Scientists and medical professionals know that people who carry extra weight around their midsections are at a higher risk of getting heart disease and diabetes. A recent study, led by Peter Havel at the University of California at Davis, put 33 overweight and obese participants on experimental diets. For the first 10 weeks, they all consumed a normal diet, but for the second 10 weeks, half the group consumed fructose for 25 percent of their calories and the other group consumed sucrose. Both groups gained an average of 3.3 pounds over the course of the study, but the group that consumed fructose added fat to their midsections, while the group that ate sucrose distributed the weight across their bodies. Havel admits that more studies should be done to confirm these findings, but the results are interesting and thought provoking.

If you avoid processed foods with added sugar (read the labels), stop adding sugar to your beverages and cereals, and limit your intake of sweet desserts, you will likely lose weight, gain a heightened sense of taste and smell that will help you enjoy other foods more, and sleep better. Consuming excessive amounts of sugar adds empty calories to your diet. If your dietary sugar is greater than 10 percent of your regular diet, you may be sacrificing more nutritious food choices that could be more satisfying as well.

Complex Carbohydrates A complex carbohydrate, or *polysaccharide*, is a chain of sugars bonded together. Although some contain more nutrients and fiber than others, all starches, such as, pasta, rice, bread, and cereals, are complex carbohydrates. Starchy vegetables, such as corn, potatoes, peas, and legumes, also contain complex carbohydrates.

Protein

Amino acids are important nutrients that play a vital role in the body's metabolic processes. Proteins consist of chains of amino acids that are broken down during digestion to provide nonessential and essential amino acids for cellular functions. The body also synthesizes proteins from these amino acids that form antibodies, structures (such as hair), hormones, and proteins that transport molecules from one part of the body to another. When you do not take in sufficient amounts of protein, your body breaks down muscle tissue to obtain it.

Fat

Fat is a very generic term for an array of compounds that are generally insoluble in water. They can exist as solids or liquids at room temperature, depending on their chemical structure, and are an important part of a healthy diet. All fats consist of fatty acids, and the properties of the fat, or lipid, depends on the type of fatty acids present. Types of fat that are solid at room temperature are generally saturated; that is, they consist of fatty acids that have no double bonds. The consumption of saturated fat leads to higher levels of LDL (bad cholesterol) in the body. Varieties of monounsaturated fat, such as olive and canola oils, have one double bond in their structures. Polyunsaturated fat has two or more double bonds. These unsaturated structures do not permit the molecules to pack as closely together, keeping the oils in liquid form.

Micronutrients

Micronutrients are the minerals and vitamins that the body requires for maintenance, energy, and growth and are needed in very small amounts. Vitamins act as catalysts for biological reactions when ingested with macronutrients, and trace minerals play a critical role in body metabolism, contributing to the synthesis of protein, fat, glycogen, and fluid balance, among others. A number of micronutrients have antioxidant properties; that is, they react with free radicals to prevent them from inflicting damage at the cellular level.

Vitamins

Vitamins are organic compounds that the human body requires in small amounts for maintaining the cells, tissues, and organs and for metabolizing the macronutrients that we consume. Although the body can chemically modify vitamins into other forms, it cannot synthesize them by itself. These essential compounds must be obtained in the diet. Vitamin C (ascorbic acid) and the B vitamins, which include thiamine, niacin, riboflavin, pyridoxine, cobalamin (B-12), pantothenic acid, and folic acid, are soluble in water. Vitamins A (retinal, retinol, and the carotenoids), D (ergocalciferol and chalecalciferol),

John Sinibaldi Sr. and John Sinibaldi Jr.

John Sinibaldi Sr. was an endurance cyclist who remained at the top of the sport for more than 75 years. He won his first race at the national level in 1928 at the age of 15 and his last national championship in 2001 when he was 91. During his cycling career, he set a time-trial record that stood for 50 years. John was a member of two U.S. Olympic cycling teams (1932 and 1936). He won 18 national titles as a masters cyclist and was inducted into the Bicycling Hall of Fame in 1997. John passed away peacefully at the age of 92 and was laid to rest wearing his favorite national championship jersey, a gold medal, and his old cycling shoes.

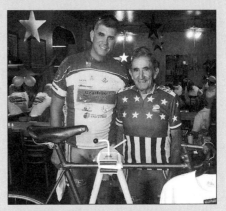

John Sinibaldi Sr. and John Sinibaldi Jr. with Sr.'s favorite 1930s steel single-speed road bike.

John Sinibaldi Jr. remembers his father fondly. "Dad rode his bike five days a week, always taking Mondays and Thursdays off. His diet was heavy on fruits and vegetables, which he grew himself organically. He never let things stress him out, and he really simplified his life when he retired. He kept his mind sharp by doing the *St. Petersburg Times* crossword puzzle until two days before he passed away. All of these certainly contributed to his long, healthy life."

Although John Jr. isn't the competitive cyclist that his father was, he appreciates his father's legacy. "I always knew my father was special but didn't appreciate how special until I was in my thirties and couldn't run anymore due to a ruptured Achilles tendon. When I started cycling, I began to spend a lot more time with him and saw how cycling kept him grounded, balanced, and focused."

John Jr. struggled with cycling for many years. His cycling was sometimes sidelined by the demands of his occupation and by a couple of bicycle accidents. One job was so stressful that he started smoking again, drinking heavily, and eating at fast food restaurants. His weight ballooned up to more than 300 pounds (136 kg), an unhealthy weight for his height of 6 feet 7 inches (2 m), and he knew he had to do something about it. He quit smoking and stuck to a diet of salads, fresh fruits, and lean meats. His weight is down to 243 (110 kg), and he hopes to reach 215 (98 kg) in another four months. He's riding 300 miles (480 km) per week, and Monday and Thursday are his easy days. John has learned to balance his cycling with running a business and raising two teenagers, both of whom are gifted intellectually and athletically. Following his father's example, he has tried to simplify his life as much as possible. He has found that committing time to ride has improved his cycling skills and has been beneficial in other areas of his life.

"I'm eating much better and taking far better care of myself. My resting heart rate is much better, my blood work is perfect, I sleep better, my headaches are gone, and my ability to recover from hard physical efforts has improved significantly."

E (tocopherols and tocotrienols), and K (phylloquinone and menaquinone) are soluble in fat. Excessive amounts of water-soluble vitamins are eliminated through urination, but excess fat-soluble vitamins can accumulate in the body. Although it's nearly impossible to overdose on vitamins obtained from food, the body can suffer from an excess of vitamin supplements.

Minerals

Linus Pauling, a two-time Nobel Prize winner, said, "You can trace every sickness, every disease, and every ailment to a mineral deficiency." Sodium and potassium, and magnesium to a lesser extent, are electrolytes that are lost during rigorous exercise through perspiration and must be replaced. Magnesium is critical for energy and for recovery after exercise, and failure to eat a diet that provides adequate amounts of this compound can contribute to accelerated fatigue, muscle cramps, and nausea. Beans, nuts, pumpkin seeds, and spinach are especially rich sources of magnesium. Sodium helps cells retain water, preventing dehydration. Hyponatremia, which occurs when sodium levels become very low, is a concern for inexperienced endurance athletes during lengthy competitions, such as an Ironman distance event, ultradistance cycling, or a marathon that takes more than four or five hours to complete. Athletes competing in endurance events such as these must include sodium in their diets, unless their physicians instruct them otherwise. Potassium is important for regulating body fluids and stabilizing muscle contractions. Many fruits and vegetables, as well as beans, milk, and yogurt are good sources of potassium. The better sports drinks usually contain all three electrolytes, making it convenient for you to replace water and minerals lost through perspiration during an endurance event.

Calcium is a mineral that is critical for bone health. Sufficient calcium can be obtained from dairy products, and endurance athletes should consume between 1,200 and 1,500 milligrams per day. Athletes who train more than six hours per week may deplete iron in their bodies. If you are not anemic, you can easily obtain the recommended 10 to 15 milligrams per day from food sources.

Another factor that contributes to anemia is excessive chromium in the body. According to the *Natural Medicine Comprehensive Database*, chromium competes with iron for binding sites on the transport protein, transferrin, which could make iron deficiencies more likely to occur. Some products on the market claim that chromium helps burn fat and develop muscle tissue; however, no reliable studies have substantiated these claims. Definite dangers are associated with excessive chromium consumption. Shortcuts for developing strong, lean bodies do not exist, so avoid gimmicks that promise otherwise.

Antioxidants

Antioxidants have an important role in minimizing cell damage during prolonged athletic activities, including cycling. The human body manufactures its own antioxidants in the form of enzymes that break down toxic peroxides

Balancing pH

PH, or potential of hydrogen, indicates acidity and alkalinity on a scale of 1 to 14. One is the most acidic, 7 is neutral, and 14 is the most alkaline. Diets that are too rich in animal products, such as red meat, milk, and eggs, will produce acid in the body, and diets that are too poor in fresh vegetables, which produce a more alkaline state, also contribute to an acidic state. Some doctors, herbalists, and nutritionists believe that pH imbalances affect the body's ability to assimilate minerals, such as calcium, potassium, sodium, and magnesium. A study at the University of California in San Francisco, which was published in the *Journal of Clinical Nutrition*, evaluated 9,000 women and determined that those with chronic acidosis were at a higher risk for loss of bone-mineral density. The body leaches calcium from the bones to balance pH, which leads to a loss of bone tissue.

Chronic, mild acidosis can also cause cardiorespiratory damage, weight gain, bladder and kidney issues, increased oxidative damage, joint pain, and accumulation of lactic acid in the muscles during athletic activity. Acidosis can be resolved by eating more alkaline-producing foods, such as fresh vegetables, citrus, almonds, sweet potatoes, and whole grains, and by choosing protein sources from animal foods that produce less acid in the body, such as fish and poultry.

into harmless compounds to be excreted. One of these enzymes, glutathione peroxidase, is bound to the mineral selenium (a micronutrient) that is essential for its activity. Other naturally occurring enzymes with antioxidant activity are catalase and superoxide dismutase, both of which serve as important defenses against oxidative cell damage. Vitamin E is a well-known scavenger of free radicals, and studies have shown that athletes who supplement their diets with vitamin E suffer less oxidative damage to their cells.

FUELING FOR TRAINING AND COMPETITION

A major limiting factor in performance is nutrition. No matter how well you have trained, your body's engine will not run properly without fuel. What you eat and drink prior to, during, and following a major expenditure of energy has a profound effect on your strength, speed, and endurance. It also greatly affects the speed and efficiency of your recovery after intense exercise.

Please keep in mind that everyone is different, and your food intake before, during, and after a race should reflect what works best for you personally. Don't wait until the day of the race to figure it out. Some athletes prefer "sports" foods, such as gels, sports beans, and bars, while others like to munch on pretzels, gummy bears, or fig bars. Be sure to establish a plan for fluid replacement. Experiment with these strategies during training so that you know how your body will respond.

The Week Before Competition

The week before competition, eat foods you are used to. Avoid new foods and those you think might cause gastrointestinal distress. While tapering your training before the event, eat carbohydrates and proteins in a 4:1 ratio, and don't limit your carbs to pasta and rice. Fruit, yogurt, and chocolate milk will add to your glycogen stores and will provide needed vitamins and minerals. You may gain weight, but don't be alarmed! A full reserve of glycogen weighs more than a pound, and 3 to 4 pounds (about 1.5 kg) of water are added during the conversion process.

Two Days Before Competition

Two days before compeition, be sure to hydrate well. I cannot stress this enough. Increase your liquid intake gradually by sipping small amount of liquids frequently throughout this period. Continue to eat as before, but include salty snacks or other electrolyte sources, including sports drinks, especially if your race will last more than a few hours, or if the weather will be hot. Performance tends to fall off when the electrolytes diminish in the body.

One Day Before Competition

The day before competition, eat a good breakfast and a bigger lunch. These are your most important meals prior to race time since they will top off your glycogen stores in time for your race. Eat familiar foods, and consume the same amount of fiber you did while you were training. Eat a good dinner, but don't overeat or eat too late. Continue hydrating.

Three to Four Hours Before Competition

Three to four hours before competition, people who suffer from prerace jitters may struggle to get food down. Eat whatever works for you for breakfast: cold cereal, oatmeal, energy bars, energy drinks, or water. It is common for athletes to experience some intestinal issues associated with prerace anxiety in the hours before the scheduled start. Drink about 17-20 ounces 2 to 3 hours prior to your event and 7-10 ounces 10-20 minutes before your start. The temperatures expected during the race and the length of the race will dictate how much you need to drink. If it is very hot, consuming a bottle of water or energy drink immediately before the start should not create a need to use the restroom since you will probably begin to lose fluids soon after you begin.

During Competition

What and how much you consume during a race depends on the length of the event and the weather conditions. Try to take in enough fluids to match what you lose; don't wait until you are thirsty. Many athletes try to consume between

500 and 1,000 milligrams of sodium for every hour they are on the bike, but excessive amounts of any electrolyte can cause nausea and vomiting. If you eat a gel or an energy bar, make sure that you also take in an appropriate amount of liquid. If the race is long, check the sodium content of your carbohydrate; some gels have insufficient amounts of sodium, so you may need to alternate your gel consumption with a sports drink or pretzels. You should already know what works best for you from your training. Do not try anything new during the race!

After Competition

After competition, eat within the first hour after you complete your event, preferably in the first 30 minutes to maximize absorption. Carbohydrate will replenish your blood sugar and glycogen stores. Protein is necessary for your body to repair any cellular damage to your muscles and to shorten your recovery time. Nut bars plus fruit, smoothies, and chocolate milk will provide carbohydrate and protein. Postrace recovery drinks are commercially available that replenish electrolytes, carbohydrate, and protein. Carbohydrate consumption should be at least one gram for each kilogram of body weight (pounds/2.2). Usually 10-20 grams of protein is enough for most cyclists. Drink fluids for the next few hours either until your weight returns to its prerace value or your urine is a pale gold and not deeply colored.

Good nutrition is mandatory to help you to perform well as an athlete and to enjoy overall good health. Eat a balanced diet that includes carbohydrate, protein, and fat, in that order. The majority of your calories should come from carbohydrates (50 to 65 percent), much of which should consist of fruits and vegetables. Limit your protein consumption (12 to 18 percent of calories) to lean meats, nuts, and low-fat dairy products. Avoid saturated fats, and include healthy fats in your diet, keeping overall fat consumption to 20 to 30 percent of your daily calories. Nutrition and hydration before, during, and following an event are very personal requirements that require experimentation during training. Try a variety of sports drinks, gels, energy bars, or other high carbohydrate food to find out which helps you maximize your performance and endurance. Establish a plan, stick to it, and don't try anything new during a race.

Preparing to Race

T.S. Eliot once said, "Only those who will risk going too far can possibly find out how far one can go." This is true, but don't sabotage a continuing interest in cycling competition by striking out too hard and too quickly. Turning your dreams of competing into solid athletic achievements requires a well-planned program with training goals to steer your course. Goals are the mileposts that mark your progress and give you interim victories that feed your competitive spirit. Success comes with a price, and greater successes come at higher costs. You must determine how much of yourself you can or want to spend.

FORMULATING REALISTIC GOALS

The longer you cycle, the more you learn about yourself. These revelations will change how you train. You must exercise reason since motivation and passion cannot make up for goals that are set too high. This experience of mine may bring some perspective.

I very much wanted to win the first Race Across America (RAAM), which in its inaugural year was known as the Great American Race, but my performance was overshadowed by a better-trained competitor. I underestimated the preparation necessary for an ultradistance race of this magnitude and finished second. The experience was so mentally and physically grueling that I never had the desire to do another RAAM. Following that hard-learned lesson, I set a more realistic and personal goal: to break the 24-hour world record for distance on a bicycle. I took a more methodical approach this time, setting interim goals and marking my progress by their achievement. Considering defeats and setbacks to be part of the maturation process, I worked, trained, and spoke with coaches, peers, and mentors. Their feedback was invaluable. It took three years and three attempts, but I broke the record, and the achievement was exhilarating and gratifyingly sweet.

Therefore, I recommend that you set realistic goals with reasonable time-frames for training. This does not exclude goals that are challenging. You will likely need to compete at the regional level before attempting a national title, or win a national title before competing for a world title. Regardless of whether your objectives are driven by competition or fitness, this methodic approach will help you better define your goals and work more efficiently to achieve them.

Identify your goals before you start training, and think of your plan as a staircase spiraling upward with increasingly challenging steps and landings that mark your interim achievements. You must consider the demands that your job and family will place on you and plan your training around them. You will undoubtedly refine your goals as you proceed with your training. I use the following approach with masters multisport and cycling athletes:

1. Evaluate the athlete's personality to determine athletic temperament.
2. Conduct quantitative physical testing to determine physiological strengths and weaknesses.
3. Compare the sport-specific parametric model with the athlete's test results.
4. Identify the athlete's strengths and weaknesses relative to sport, lifestyle, environment, and personal relationships. My coaching experience indicates that relationships directly affect an athlete's performance.
5. Develop a coaching strategy that is consistent with the preceding guidelines.

In addition, effective coaches provide their clients with a training manual that supplements the coaching efforts and includes reference material for the following activities:

- *Training off the bike*: Include flexibility routines, strengthening exercises, and general fitness workouts.
- *Road workouts*: Include time trials, hill repeats, and interval training.
- *Track workouts*: These should be based on individual-sport focus and availability of facilities.
- *Cycling techniques*: Include climbing, descending, cornering, braking, shifting, and riding in a pack.
- *Cycling tactics*: These should be specific to training objectives, such as fitness and type of competition.

- *Fitting*: Include a thorough setup that is based on the application, such as road and track workouts, time trials, and mountain biking.

If you work without a personal coach, many cycling and triathlon clubs have coached workouts, but they will not be geared toward you as an individual. It will be up to you to honestly assess your temperament, strengths, and weakness before beginning a program. You may be able to find information to assist you online, but it is far more expedient to have a professional assessment before embarking on a program by yourself.

I worked with a client whose training goals became completely absorbed by the formidable challenges of competing in the RAAM. His support crew was in place and his financial backing was close to finalization. Unfortunately, he had not balanced his training with the rest of his responsibilities, and he was haunted by guilt because of the long hours he spent in the saddle. He felt defeated before he had even competed in the event. When training is no longer fun, it becomes drudgery. Motivation slips away, widening the gap between you and your goal. Looking too hard at the big picture can be intimidating. A journey such as this begins with the first stroke of the pedal. Interim goals are signposts of success along the way. Take it one step at a time.

CREATING A PERIODIZATION PLAN

You have set your short- and long-term goals, and now you are ready to plan your training. Periodization is a concept based on a scientific model created by Hans Selye, a Canadian endocrinologist, whose work has been used by the sports community since the 1950s. His general adaptation syndrome is based on the body's physiological response to stress, which he categorized into three stages:

1. *Alarm.* Physical stress is initially experienced by the body.
2. *Resistance.* The body adapts to the applied stress.
3. *Exhaustion.* Physical recovery from the applied stress is inadequate, and the physical output of the body decreases.

Eustress, Selye's name for positive stress, causes the body to increase muscular strength, speed, and endurance; *distress*, or negative stress, causes cellular damage to muscles and joints and can compromise the immune system. The goal of periodic training is to keep the body in the resistance stage and to avoid slipping into exhaustion. After the body recovers from applied stress, it is better equipped to deal with increased demands. The applied stress can then be elevated in intensity or duration. Selye's model allows athletes to break the training process into bite-sized pieces that maximize the opportunities for successful results:

- *Sport-specific testing.* Use primary metrics, including heart rate, mph, wattage, and rpm.

- *Sport-specific training.* Use the coaching model to create a training plan that is driven by goals.
- *Goals.* Establish milestones and interim goals and refine them as you monitor your progress.
- *Development of recognition and reaction skills.* Sharpen your competitive edge by practicing racing drills and competing in races.
- *Evaluation and refinement.* Evaluate your performance and adjust your training plan accordingly.

If the body slips into an exhausted state from overtraining, there are a number of symptoms that may be observed, including:

- A feeling of deep fatigue and a lack of energy
- A general feeling of achiness or pain in the joints and muscles
- An abrupt decline in performance
- Inability to sleep
- Headaches
- A compromised immune system (more frequent illnesses)
- Feeling irritable or out of sorts
- Feeling depressed
- Lack of enthusiasm for cycling
- Loss of appetite
- More frequent injuries
- An obsessive need to train

If you suspect that you may have "overtraining syndrome," take a few days to rest, drink plenty of water, and eat a nutritious diet. Your body will thank you and reward you with improved performance.

Every aspect of your life, from the weather to your responsibilities, dictates the pace and quality of your training. The time frame of your program is measured in weeks (microcycle), months (mesocycle), and years (macrocycle). A macrocycle may be as short as one year for someone preparing for an ultradistance event or as long as eight years for an aspiring Olympian. Active recovery is desirable in a successful training plan, which schedules intermittent days of low-intensity cycling, swimming, running, or similar activities. Management of the different elements of training, such as strength and endurance, must be separated from other elements of the program to obtain maximum benefits.

Periodization provides peaks and valleys in the intensity and duration of your training and varies the types of exercises you do. Without variation, your body adapts to the stresses placed on it, and the benefits you receive from your efforts decline with time. Without adequate rest, your body cannot recover from the stress of training and become stronger. Each person has individual physical

Rusko's Exhaustion Test

Studies done by Finnish researcher Heikki Rusko indicate that there may be a way to determine if you are approaching Selye's exhaustion stage. Rusko's study population consisted of elite Finnish cross-country skiers during an intense 13 weeks of training. He developed a simple evaluation routine that he called an *orthostatic test*. The test was conducted on athletes at the same time each day.

The participants were asked to lie quietly for a period of 10 minutes, during which their heart rates were monitored and recorded. They stood up, and after 15 seconds and again between 90 and 120 seconds, their heart rates were recorded. Most of the athletes recorded very consistent heart rates from day to day (for example, 60 beats per minute (bpm) resting, 95 bpm after 15 seconds of standing, and 80 bpm after 90 to 120 seconds of standing). Rusko found that athletes who were showing symptoms of overtraining exhibited elevated heart rates after standing. For example, the heart rates measured 90 to 120 seconds after standing were between 90 and 95 bpm, compared to the 80 bpm of those who were not overtrained. Rusko also found that the rise in heart rate gradually occurred over a four-week period, indicating that athletes can modify training protocol if an increase in standing heart rate is observed over time.

Over the years, I have monitored my heart rate upon waking in the morning. According to research I did for this book, this practice is unreliable. Rusko's test is easily done with a heart monitor and is considered to yield values that are more credible; however, additional data is needed to further substantiate these findings.

limits, age-related or otherwise, and training and racing experience, so their programs must be formulated accordingly. A traditional periodization plan allows for higher mileage with lower output in the off-season and shorter mileage that is more intense during racing season. Peaking is a function of tapering the program slightly as important events come up. Tapering, as the term implies, is the gradual reduction of mileage, duration, and intensity of workouts. Avoid the mindset that you are being lazy during this process. Avoid a regimented program of inflexible training exercises that you follow for interminable periods with pedantic discipline and little or no diversion. These plans do not allow for self-analysis, growth, or a change of direction, and they may lead to burnout and a failure to make real progress.

Computer-driven training programs that follow rigid and impersonal guidelines are the bane of creative training. They prevent aspiring athletes from exploring their true potential. For example, an aspiring road racer may turn out to be a natural time trialist or to have a talent for circuit racing. Dynamic diversion is an exceedingly preferable alternative to the one-size-fits-all program structure that some well-meaning coaches promote. A more realistic and enjoyable periodization program that allows for spontaneity will achieve better long-term results.

Seasonal Training

Living in southern California or other warm locations that allow for year-round cycling may appear to offer a big advantage. However, environments with inclement weather merely change the format of the training, not its quality. Training in a harsher climate requires you to focus on indoor-cycling workouts and strength training and to increase your intensity. Regardless of the season, riding every day can be great, but it can also be a dead end if the training loses variety and becomes monotonous. Most of my clients who live in harsher climates and cannot ride outdoors are comfortable with a straightforward program of building and recovery with off-season diversions, such as cross-country skiing, snowshoeing, indoor swimming, indoor cycling, climbing, and ice-skating. Consequently, their periodization components last longer and involve a gradual buildup of conditioning. Winter workouts should include interval training and a variety of intensities. Athletes can prevent the loss of cycling skills and sport-specific strength by incorporating short, intense leg-speed drills into their winter training.

Many things can influence how and where you can train, such as the environment and your individual needs. The structure of your training program depends on the following factors:

- *Weather conditions.* The type of climate that you live in affects the duration of your periodization cycles.

- *Cycling event.* Your training will depend on whether you're racing or riding and on the types of cycling events you want to compete or participate in, such as time trials, road races or rides, or track, mountain-bike, BMX, or cyclo-cross races. Consider also whether your goals include shorter distances or ultradistance events.

- *Your micro-, meso-, and macro- (short-term, intermediate, and long-term) training goals.* These dictate the amount of mileage you must ride, as well as the other components of your training.

- *Age.* Older athletes require recovery days that are longer or more frequent.

- *Available time.* Demanding schedules necessitate shorter, more-intense workouts.

The decision to begin a program is usually accompanied by a strong desire to get started. Most of my regular clients are excited about starting a new plan, and they typically begin their training programs after an active-rest period in the early fall that lasts from three to six weeks. I encourage participating in a number of psychological exercises and using motivational tapes to help with mental preparation for the upcoming season.

Ralph Waldo Emerson once said, "Make the most of yourself, for that is all there is of you." Some of my most successful clients take this message to heart. Here is another Emerson quotation that speaks to masters athletes: "We need not count a man's years until there is nothing left to count." Your attitude as you approach your training can have a profound effect on the outcome. Mental preparation is a vital part of successful periodization training.

Autumn

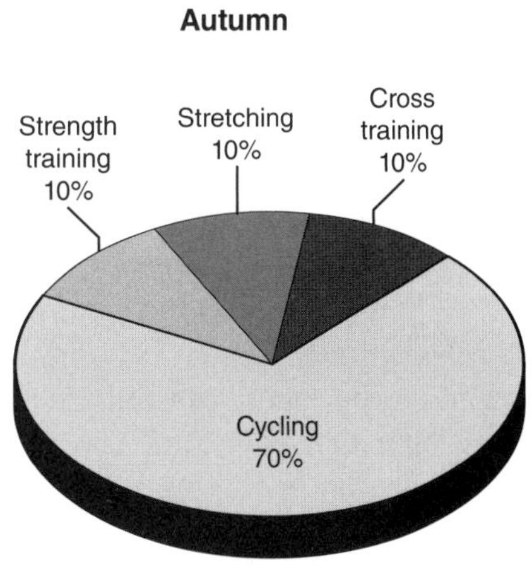

The best time to start a new training program is in the autumn when the traditional cycling season is ending (see figure 8.1). This is an excellent time to evaluate the efficiency of your previous training program and to take stock of your physical status in terms of flexibility, strength, and speed. How well did you achieve your goals during the previous season? Where were you deficient? Were you plagued by pain or injuries?

During autumn, your weekly road mileage should drop off gradually. By winter, it should be limited to one long base ride, usually during the weekend. If you add a second base day, it should be midweek. Orient your training at the gym or at home toward balancing flexibility and core strength. Your goal is to have body symmetry in terms of strength and flexibility to decrease the risk of injury.

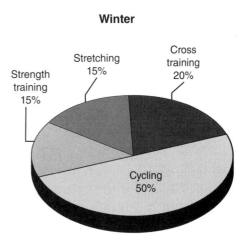

Autumn

Strength training 10%
Stretching 10%
Cross training 10%
Cycling 70%

Figure 8.1 Autumn periodization.

Winter

The winter months are ideal for focusing on strength training (see figure 8.2). You should do flexibility and core workouts five or six times each week. General and sport-specific strength workouts are designed to address your specific needs. On the trainer, add single-leg and leg-speed drills to remind your muscles that their newly acquired strength is for turning the cranks. Maintain conditioning off the bike by running, preferably on asphalt roads or dirt trails, to keep your muscles supple. You may add plyometric exercises in small doses.

Winter

Strength training 15%
Stretching 15%
Cross training 20%
Cycling 50%

Figure 8.2 Winter periodization.

Progressive resistance training (see chapter 4) will advance from a phase of basic development with lighter weights and more repetitions (two or three sets of 10 to 12 repetitions), to a phase of strength and endurance training with light to moderate weights and a gradual increase in resistance (two or three sets of 12 to 14 repetitions) once or twice a week. Each phase should last four to six weeks. As winter progresses, you will enter the power phase, doing six to eight repetitions at 85 to 90 percent of maximum weight in concentric motions that are explosive, yet controlled. Follow these with slow, eccentric returns one day per week. In addition to this high-intensity workout, spend one day per week adding two or three sets of 12 to 14 repetitions at 65 percent of the maximum weight you can handle. At this time, if weather permits, spend one or two longer days each week riding on the road.

Spring

Spring is the season for focusing on sport-specific training (see figure 8.3). Focus on maintaining strength conditioning rather than building it, adding more repetitions and decreasing weight for muscle tone. Your saddle time will shift from longer base rides to a variety of shorter workouts. This is the ideal time for single-leg drills, which are used to assess the balance of leg flexibility and strength, leg-speed workouts to promote faster pedal turnover, and progressive stall-outs and hill repeats (explained later in this chapter), which move strength training out of the gym and onto the bike.

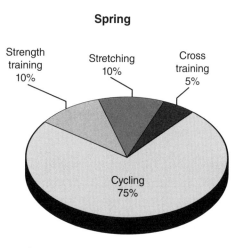

Figure 8.3 Spring periodization.

Continue running once or twice per week for shorter distances, emphasizing hills. A 15-minute, low-intensity workout will help keep your body weight in check. At this time, fill out your racing calendar and shift your training to target the closest event. If possible, ride the course at least one time before the event to learn about road conditions and the severity of various features, such as turns, climbs, and descents.

Summer

During the summer months, maintain your form and fitness level (see figure 8.4). It's hot, and you're in peak form. You will not do yourself any favors by hammering out road miles in the quest of a race-ready body. Although you are currently focusing on competition or other goal events, rest days and active recovery are essential to prevent overtraining syndrome. Remember Selye's general adaptation syndrome. Failure to recover adequately may produce physiological and psychological symptoms that can turn a promising season

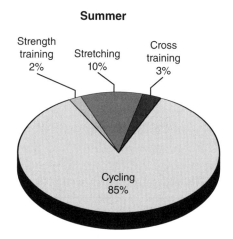

Figure 8.4 Summer periodization.

Al Whaley

Anyone familiar with the history of cycling will recognize the name Marshall Walter Taylor, better known as Major Taylor, who was the world's first African-American sports champion. Major Taylor's achievements were remarkable even by today's standards, but in the late 1800s, his successes were earned while fighting battles on and off the track.

In 1997, nearly 100 years after Major Taylor won his first world cycling championship, another African-American cyclist made history by winning the first of 14 world cycling championships in match sprinting, which had been Major Taylor's specialty. Al Whaley not only resembles the Major in stature, but he also rides like him. Vic Copeland, one of Al's toughest masters rivals, noted that Al is incredibly quick with an almost feminine quality in the way he sprints.

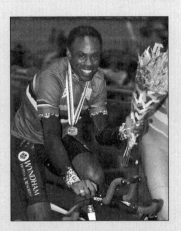

Al Whaley, winner of more than a dozen world masters sprints and 1-kilometer races.

Published reports of Taylor's style note similar characteristics: Both riders favored small gears and a high cadence, and both men had an abundance of fast-twitch muscle fibers.

Al credits his success in cycling to his coach, Bill Edwards, who is an accomplished cyclist with a solid coaching resumé. "Without Coach Bill, I wouldn't be the person or the athlete I have become over the years. I look at him as the jeweler and myself as the gem. A jeweler can see the diamond in the rough when everyone else sees a stone. Bill prepared me to become the athlete I had only imagined I could ever be. The results of his training methods were very apparent after he became my coach. Since he started coaching me in the mid 1990s, I have been blessed to win more races than I can count, not including the second and third place finishes along the way."

Al is very involved with challenged athletes and received the Olympic Spirit Award at the 2000 Paralympic Games held in Sydney, Australia. He and his tandem teammate, Pam Fernandez, also won gold and silver medals there. They set a new world and Olympic-Paralympic record in the 1-kilometer time trial with a time of 1:08:996, making them the first tandem cycling team in U.S. history to win the gold medal at an Olympic event.

As Al has aged, he feels that he has gotten stronger and faster with less training. However, it takes him longer to recover from some events. Once he discovered that his mental preparation is every bit as important as being physically ready, he started winning on a more consistent basis. Al took a few years off from competition and is just now returning to the sport. "When I was fit and racing, staying up front was the best place to be. Now, I find it harder to do that since my fitness level isn't what it once was. My current strategy is to stay in the middle of the peloton."

Cycling has had a huge effect on Al's life, and he is very appreciative of the experiences he has enjoyed with the sport. "I have met so many people I never would have met otherwise, and I've had the opportunity to travel to many different countries and learn about the diverse cultures that exist all over the world. At the same time, I have been able to race my bike and enjoy doing the thing I love so much."

into a disappointing one. Listen to your body's signals. If you experience mild but continual leg soreness, muscular and joint pain, a sudden decline in performance, loss of appetite, insomnia, an increase in the frequency of illnesses, more injuries, or a loss of enthusiasm for the sport, your body may need more rest than you're giving it. If you are experiencing one or more of these symptoms, take a few days off, drink plenty of fluids, and eat a healthy diet.

The general principles of periodization previously outlined constitute a process that is integral to achieving your cycling goals. Within that framework, you will obtain the best results by systematically building your cycling skills, flexibility, and strength through a variety of moderate and intense training workouts that are followed by periods of active recovery. Active recovery is vital for you to obtain maximum benefits from your training. Without it, you will overtrain, fail to achieve results, and burn out mentally and physically.

Cardiorespiratory Training

Off-season diversions, like running, should follow the format of moderate, high, and then mild intensity in order for them to pay big dividends for overall fitness. Even in the midst of a busy competition season or general fitness training, you can slide into a funk from repetitive training. When this occurs or you feel it coming on, mix some other kinds of training into your plan.

Running up hills at low output improves cardio capacity and range, bone density, and overall strength. Depending on your competitive schedule, adding running to your training can be valuable throughout the year. Run on trails or asphalt when you can, avoiding concrete surfaces to lessen the impact.

Hiking is a great sport for active recovery and is a good way to enjoy outdoor scenery. It's a nice diversion from a stagnated regimen and a great tool for overall body conditioning. In 1976, I won the Atlantic City '76, America's biggest single-day race, following a four-day hike in the Green Mountains of Vermont. After a grueling series of races or intense training, varying your activities can improve your performance by changing muscle-firing patterns and by allowing the active recovery of muscles primarily used for cycling.

Flexibility

Flexibility training should be a daily component in an effective program year-round (see chapter 4 for more information). It is an integral part of every masters workout regimen. As we age, blood flow and transfer of synovial fluid to the joints decrease, compounding the ravages of aging. By including flexibility exercises into your daily routine, you can maintain or improve your range of motion and reduce your risk of injury.

Strength

Once your body is balanced in terms of flexibility, strengthening should be your next priority. Strength training should advance in intensity during the off-season but should be used at reduced levels during the active season to maintain muscle tone and bone mass. Core strengthening should be addressed year round since a strong core is a prerequisite for strong cycling (see chapter 4 for more information).

The following table includes each of the four seasons and outlines the type of activity that is recommended along with the suggested frequency and duration of training for each component. A table of seasonal training options is also included to show you how to vary your workouts for each season. Pop in an optional activity when time allows, and have fun with it!

Table 8.1   Recommendations for Seasonal Activities

Activity	Time (hours)
Autumn	
Cardio (easy)	1.5-2.5 hrs.
Flexibility	2 hrs.
Strength	2.5 hrs. (full body)
Cardio (moderate)	2-3 hrs. (2 hrs. cycling)
Cardio (intense)	0.5 hrs.
Winter	
Cardio (easy)	1.5-2.5 hrs. (trainer)
Flexibility	2 hrs.
Strength	3 hrs. (cycling-specific and core exercises)
Cardio (moderate)	5-6 hrs. (4 hrs. cycling)
Cardio (intense)	1 hr.
Spring	
Cardio (easy)	1.75-2.75 hrs. (trainer/road)
Flexibility	1.75 hrs.
Strength	1 hr. (core/stabilizers)
Cardio (moderate)	5-6 hrs.
Cardio (intense)	2-3 hrs. (training/racing)
Summer	
Cardio (easy)	3-5 hrs.
Flexibility	1.5 hrs.
Strength	0.5 hr (core/stabilizers)
Cardio (moderate)	4-6 hrs.
Cardio (intense)	1.75-2.5 hrs. (training/racing)

Table 8.2   Options for Seasonal Activities

Cardio (easy)	Cardio (moderate)	Cardio (intense)	Flexibility	Strength
Cycling in zones 1 and 2	Hypoxic intervals (see page 129)	Hill repeats (see page 131)	Stretching	Strength training
Walking	Swimming	Time trial (club)	Yoga	Core training
Hiking*	Cycling in zones 2 and 3	Cross-country skiing	Pilates	Progressive stall-outs (see page 128)
Dancing	Running*	Indoor cycling (anaerobic intervals)	Gymnastics	Power climbing
Single-leg drills	Indoor cycling	Jump rope	Exercise ball	Plyometric training
	Hiking*	Cardio kickboxing		Climbing (rock or wall)
	Single-leg drills	Leg-speed drills		
		Running*		

*Intensity depends on pace and terrain.

Periodization Training

Instead of providing you with the same, tired training exercises you often see in many plans, I would like to present some effective workouts that represent cutting-edge training techniques.

Progressive Stall-Outs

Progressive stall-outs are a training technique developed by Bill Edwards, a successful cycling coach with an engineering background whose racing and coaching experience spans more than 60 years. Use an indoor power-training system with a power meter, such as the CompuTrainer, with your road bike. Follow these instructions for the progressive stall-out drill:

1. Calibrate your power meter for tire friction according to your unit's manual.

2. Program your course with a short 40- to 50-meter hill. I programmed my system with a 5 percent drop, immediately followed by a 17 percent rise.

3. Warm up for 15 minutes.

4. On your first effort, use an easy gear, such as 53 by 21. Increase your cadence to a target rpm, such as 80 to 120 rpm for roadies or 150 to 160 rpm for sprinters. Ride through the course; it should be easy.

5. For each subsequent effort, gear up a single cog at a time until you are struggling to maintain your targeted rpm to finish the course. You should be able to complete four to six efforts with five minutes of active recovery (easy pedaling) between efforts.

Check the number of pedal strokes needed to climb the hill. If you are taking more than 6 to 10 strokes, shorten the course. An overly long course will prevent you from maximizing the intensity of your workout. Be sure to save courses during the rest periods, and evaluate them with your system's software, if available. Once you have trained long enough to achieve your targeted output of sustainable power, maintain your fitness level each week with a single workout of one or two efforts at the same level of intensity that you achieved at the end of the program. Missing a week, however, can result in declined power output. If you cannot avoid this situation, and you are struggling to complete 6 to 10 pedal strokes without breaking form, you can recover your previous fitness level by repeating the program for two to three weeks.

As with any type of intense training, recovery from this program is critical. Microtears occur in the muscle cells during training, and the process of cell repair increases your strength. It can take a few days to recover. If you can stand it, taking an ice bath immediately after the workout may accelerate the recovery process.

Hypoxic Intervals

Training under hypoxic conditions has been a very controversial topic. In the medical sense, hypoxia is the limited availability of oxygen to part or all of the body. In hypoxic training, you hold your breath during an interval; for example, you might hold your breath for 15 seconds during a one-minute interval of pedaling at zone 2 (or higher for more advanced cyclists). Some sources maintain that hypoxic-interval training stimulates the body into an adaptation similar to that of high-altitude acclimatization. In response to the hypoxic environment, the body produces erythropoietin (EPO), a hormone that controls erythropoiesis, or the production of red blood cells. EPO stimulates the production of blood-cell precursors, protects blood cells from apoptosis (cell death), and helps wounds heal. EPO that is exogenous, or produced outside the body, has been used to stimulate growth of red blood cells for patients with anemia.

Proponents cite controlled studies which indicate that hypoxic training may reduce the adverse effects of hypoxia on the autonomic nervous system by enhancing ventilatory drive (breathing controlled by the autonomic nervous system) and by increasing the efficiency of the body's use of oxygen. Swimmers, who regularly control their breathing while performing, have used hypoxic-interval training for more than 20 years since low-frequency breathing patterns can allow for more speed. Sheila Taormina, a former Olympic swimmer and triathlete, had the fastest swim spilt (1.5 km) in the 2000 Olympic women's triathlon. She finished in at 19:02:78 by breathing every three strokes. Hypoxic intervals also help swimmers feel more comfortable with the physiological response to oxygen deprivation.

Opponents of hypoxic training refer to controlled studies that compare athletes who have trained under hypoxic conditions with those training at sea level. Some studies have found no significant difference between the test and control groups in $\dot{V}O_2$max, speed, or O_2 saturation of the arterial blood. Hypoxic conditions exist at high altitudes, in hypobaric chambers, or with a number of commercially available hypoxicators, such as the CVAC (cyclic variations in altitude conditioning). The CVAC is an environment that produces dynamic changes in air pressure to simulate variations in altitude. Instead of spending a restless night in an altitude tent, spend 20 minutes in a CVAC pod for similar results. I find that holding my breath during exertion also has a similar effect. My training clients perform variations of the following routine on a trainer or rollers before a workout or race:

1. Pedal for 2 to 3 minutes.
2. Hold your breath while pedaling to reach the heart rate for zone 2 or 3 for 15 seconds.
3. Resume breathing for the remaining 45 seconds.
4. Repeat this cycle five to eight times.

I have personally found that this routine effectively warms up the muscles without overtaxing them, and I have received positive feedback from all of my training clients. However, be forewarned: Holding your breath for prolonged periods or engaging in hypoxic training is potentially dangerous. Discontinue the practice if you experience dizziness, disorientation, or any other unusual physical symptoms.

Single-Leg Drills

When pedaling, one leg tends to dominate the other. This inefficient practice creates an imbalance in the stress applied to the body. Single-leg drills are an important element of training to help both legs develop pedaling strength. You will learn to apply equal pressure to both pedals, thereby increasing the efficiency of each stroke and reducing the risk for injury.

1. Warm up with 5 to 10 minutes of spinning, gradually increasing speed to 60 to 80 rpm.
2. Pedal with one leg for 15 seconds, alternating between left and right twice. Pedal with both legs for 15 seconds at 60 to 80 rpm.
3. Pedal for 30 seconds with the left leg, then for 30 seconds with the right leg. Repeat this cycle once, then pedal with both legs for 30 seconds.
4. Pedal for 45 seconds with the left leg, then for 45 seconds with the right leg. Repeat this cycle once, then pedal with both legs for 45 seconds.
5. Pedal for one minute with the left leg, then for one minute with the right leg. Repeat this cycle once, then pedal with both legs for one minute.

If, at any point during the workout, you find that you cannot turn the cranks, stop and drop back to the previous level. This drill increases strength and coordination of the hip flexors, which have a large effect on pedal-stroke efficiency.

Leg-Speed Drills

Varying your cadence is a great way to recruit more muscles and to enhance muscle-firing patterns. Rapid spinning promotes nourishment of the capillary cells. I recently did a training ride with a group of fit, ultradistance specialists. I was amazed to see that none of them could respond to aggressive attacks or fast surges. It became clear to me that aerobic training that is dominated by a middle-gear tempo fails to develop fast-twitch muscle fibers. Leg speed is an important factor for aggressive, competitive cycling. Here is the perfect 30-minute workout for those who do not race but want to be competitive on weekend group rides:

1. Warm up slowly for 10 to 15 minutes, gradually building rpm.
2. Pedal for 1 minute in S-3 (small ring, cog number counted from largest cog) at 90 rpm.
3. Pedal for 1 minute in S-3 at 100 rpm.
4. Pedal for 1 minute in S-3 at 110 rpm.
5. Pedal easily for 2 minutes to recover.
6. Pedal for one minute in S-4 at 100 rpm. For the last 10 seconds, accelerate aggressively in the saddle in L-4 (large ring, cog number counted from largest cog).
7. Repeat this sequence three times.
8. Pedal easily for 5 minutes to recover.

Hill Repeats

Hill repeats are done in late winter toward the end of the power phase of strength training. These short workouts are suitable if the weather is still cold. If you have a programmable trainer, you can do this workout indoors although you usually experience the feeling of climbing much better when on the road. This type of workout gives you the ability to tolerate high workloads and to produce explosive pedaling motions that can give you a strategic advantage in racing and can improve your overall performance.

The hill gradient is specific to individual conditioning, training, and power. Most of my clients use a grade of 6 to 9 percent and a distance between 300 and 400 meters. Before starting, warm up for 15 to 25 minutes indoors on a trainer or rollers, or outdoors if weather allows, and then do the following:

1. In the saddle, pedal with a fast turnover (80 to 90 rpm) using a lighter gear (moderate).

2. In the saddle, pedal with a slow turnover (30 to 50 rpm) in a big gear (moderate to intense).

3. Ride at a hard race pace (70 to 85 rpm) in an intermediate gear and include sets both in and out of the saddle (intense).

4. Repeat the preceding set until your heart rate fails to recover normally or your wattage drops off. Allow two to three minutes for active recovery between sets. For example, do a quick turnover while pedaling down the grade you just rode up.

I enjoy designing effective training programs that will get my clients to the finish line of a race or into good cycling condition. Athletes should have a solid understanding of the key training components, including how and when they should be implemented. They should also have a strong mental attitude when approaching training to ensure that their efforts yield the desired results down the road.

Strategies for Every Event

In competition, you may take your pick from many types of rides and races. These fun and masters-friendly competitive events will challenge you and will give your training purpose. Centuries, cross-state rides, time trials, road races, track racing, criteriums, cyclo-cross, mountain bike rides and competitions, and triathlons demand their own training strategies and racing tactics. You have now gained a better understanding of the general training process and have begun to practice your technical skills, so it's time to put that training to good use.

INDIVIDUAL TIME TRIALS

If you're a novice, time trials are safer and less scary than pack riding. They also allow you to develop your power as you work on your group-riding skills elsewhere. Since they are solo events, you don't have to worry about drafting, and any pressure to perform is self-imposed. The bike split in triathlons is essentially a time trial because time penalties are imposed for violations and drafting is not allowed unless you're a pro. Time trials emphasize sustained power output, which requires a well-developed aerobic capacity derived from anaerobic training. They can range in distance from a few miles to 40 kilometers. You will soon discover how hard you can ride before you reach your mental and physical limits. You are out there on your own with nowhere to hide. These events can be painfully intense, but getting a PR (personal record) is a very gratifying and exhilarating experience.

General Equipment

The range of cycling events means many types of equipment. Most riders use road, track, and off-road bikes. Any major purchase requires thoughtful consideration. Wait to buy the newest model until you have competed or participated in organized races or rides. You can upgrade your equipment once you have a better idea of your interests. When you're starting to compete, equipment isn't as important as attitude and preparation.

Some genres of cycling have specific equipment requirements. If you plan to do track training or racing, choose a single-speed, fixed-gear bike without brakes. For off-road cycling, choose a mountain bike with low gears, knobby tires, and suspension to make rough rides more comfortable. Choose a standard road bike for road racing, criteriums, triathlons, and time trials. You can easily fit it with aero bars and aerodynamic wheels if needed.

Helmet

A quality helmet that fits well and is ANSI-approved is essential for protecting your head. Helmets come in a large array of styles, colors, and prices. Although cheaper helmets offer sufficient protection, helmets that are more expensive are superior since they are lighter and allow for better ventilation. Wear a skullcap underneath your helmet or a facemask for cold or freezing temperatures.

Shoes

Buy the best shoes you can afford for optimal comfort, durability, and functionality. Good shoes help you efficiently transfer energy to the pedals. Different designs exist for road biking, triathlon, and mountain biking. Make sure they fit well and provide sufficient room in the toe box. Remember that feet can swell in hot weather.

Gloves

Gloves protect and cushion the hands, reducing the risk of nerve damage from long-term pressure against the handlebars and guarding against severe abrasions during a crash.

Cycling Shorts

Padded cycling shorts that fit close to the body allow for aerodynamics and increased comfort during long rides. High-quality shorts last longer, look better, fit better, and are more comfortable. Do not wear underwear with cycling shorts! If you must have something underneath them, choose a liner without seams to avoid chafing.

Preparing for Time Trials

The best way to become proficient at time trials is to do a lot of them. It's best to start out with shorter TTs, such as 15 to 25 minutes once a week, and move on from there. Many triathlon clubs incorporate time trials into their weekly training schedules, so you have options other than an actual race while learning. Do you ride better with a higher cadence and smaller gears or with a slower

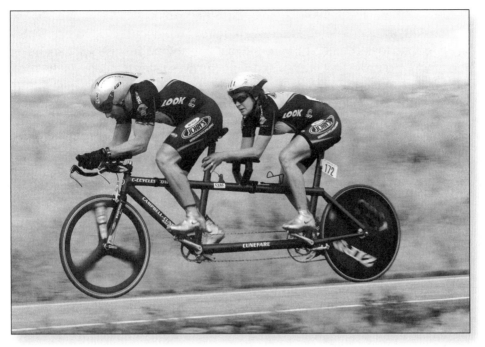

Bryan Van Vleet and Susan Cooper on the tandem bike in perfect aero form, winning the Mixed Elite National Championships.

cadence and bigger gears? This is something you will learn as you train. Big chain rings are commonly used in time trials.

Time trialing requires speed and endurance. An excellent training exercise is to ride high-output intervals of two, four, and six minutes, allowing enough recovery time in between to make a good effort on the next interval. A road that is flat or slightly rolling is ideal for this kind of training. When your heart rate can no longer return to the rate seen in earlier recovery periods, it's time to ride gently. Training with a heart-rate monitor makes this easier, and power meters show drops in wattage that indicate it's time to cruise. During your training session, try to hold your rpm between 75 and 95 for the duration. Toward the end of the workout, be sure to note the following:

1. Your optimal rpm range and how this value varies due to course terrain, wind, and fatigue.
2. Your sustainable heart-rate zones.
3. Your approximate sustainable wattage for the conditions, if you're using a power meter. Your heart rate and wattage should rise during the final three to five minutes of your race.

This exercise will help you determine both the most effective rpm range for you and the optimal gear for maintaining it. You must practice this under a variety of conditions.

You should also become familiar with the turnaround technique; that is, negotiating the U-turn at the halfway point of an out-and-back course. There are two ways to negotiate a turnaround, but the method you use will depend on the amount of room that is available. One involves using the cone as the apex of your turn and utilizing the entire lane to complete it. This works best if there is a lot of room to maneuver in. However, if the lane is narrow, you may want to ride closer to the right of the cone, brake hard, and turn, resuming your pedal strokes as soon as you can. Set out a cone or half-full water bottle in an empty parking lot or long, straight driveway. Practice your turnarounds slowly at first and pick up your speed as you become more comfortable with the maneuver. You may lose a little time with a turnaround that is more cautious, but not as much as you will if you crash.

Aerodynamics in Individual Time-Trials

Racing in a time trial means that you are literally on your own. Drafting is not a factor, so aerodynamics are critical for this kind of event. You can reduce the drag of wind resistance by choosing proper equipment, bike position, and clothing.

Equipment for Time Trials

If you are preparing for your first time trial or triathlon, just do it on a standard road bike. If you want to spend money on equipment, start out by bolting aero bars to your road bike. They come in many shapes, sizes, materials, and prices, and are advantageous because they put you in an aerodynamic posture on the bike. Your next priority should be investing in a pair of aerodynamic racing wheels, which range from wheels with aerodynamic rims and spokes to disc wheels for the rear. If you have to choose between the two, forego the disc wheels, which are problematic in crosswinds.

If you are ready to take to take a serious plunge into financing your chosen sport, look for bikes with carbon-fiber frames that are more steeply angled specifically for time trials. These light and aerodynamic bikes are stiff, so that the power applied to the pedals isn't absorbed by the frame or the bicycle's components. Instead, the energy goes directly to the drive train to give you more speed. The lighter, stiffer, and more aerodynamic the bike is, the faster it will be. These machines can be outfitted with the racing wheels of your choice and, of course, aerobars. An aerodynamic helmet, skin suit, and booties complete a professional-looking ensemble.

Another consideration for the serious competitor is tubular tires, or "sew-ups." Instead of having an inner tube inside a casing with two edges that are popped into the rim to seal them (clinchers), tubular tires consist of an inner tube that is completely encased in a treaded, rubberized covering that is sewn together and then glued to the rim with a contact cement. The installation can be messy and time-consuming, but there are benefits. These tires are lighter than clinchers, and so are the rims they are attached to. The materials the tires are composed of contribute to a smoother ride, and they offer more stability should a puncture occur. You can carry a pre-glued spare for a quick changeout if you do suffer a puncture.

If you really want to increase your speed, make sure you are professionally fit to your bike to maximize your power output. Also, obtaining a good training program from a qualified cycling coach is an excellent way to improve your overall performance. At the risk of sounding redundant, you don't need to buy extreme equipment unless you are competing at an elite or professional level, where fractions of a second can separate you from your competition. Fabian Cancellara, winner of the opening time-trial stage of the 2009 Tour de France, rode a bike that weighed an astonishingly heavy 16.8 pounds (7.6 kg) with a rear disc wheel that weighed nearly 2 pounds (1 kg)! In contrast, the late Art Longsjo, the first Olympic athlete to compete on a winter team as a speed skater and on a summer team as a cyclist, entered and won his first bike race wearing black swim trunks, a white T-shirt, and street shoes. The motor (you) and its preparation are far more important than the machine or your attire.

Bike Positioning for Time Trials

Aerodynamics means more than simply minimizing frontal area and the flow of air around the rider and bike. You should also minimize the creation of excessive turbulence and drag, which cause significant power loss at the pedals, as the air separates from the rear of the bike. This requires a compromise between aerodynamics and power. You want to be as aero as possible without losing biomechanical efficiency. The ability to use your available muscular power

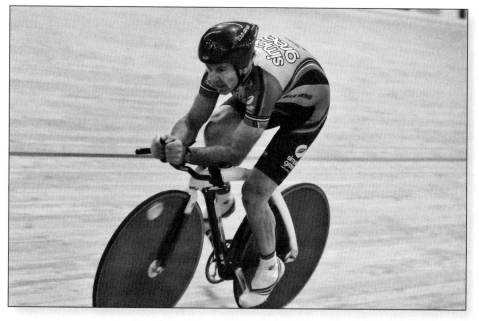

Kenny Fuller in aero position.

depends on your position. Any improvements in aerodynamics require time in the saddle to adjust since your muscles must retrain in order to fire efficiently. Finding a low profile, aerodynamic position that you can comfortably maintain without compromising key muscle groups for the duration of your event is a formidable goal. Keep your body and head as low as possible to enhance airflow, but make sure you can see the course. Don't make the mistake of being too aerodynamic. It is surprising how many Ironman triathletes cannot maintain their positions for the full 112-mile (180 km) bike split. The distance of the race will dictate how aero you go.

Strategies for Time Trial

Pacing in a time trial is all about developing a strong mental discipline and utilizing your training effectively. It's you against the clock. Knowing that you have trained properly for your event will give you confidence. Knowing the course before you enter a race will give you even more. Climbing in a time trial will push you beyond your anaerobic threshold as you maintain the momentum necessary for a good finish. When you are racing on flat terrain, find the sweet spot between riding at your anaerobic threshold and exceeding it.

Before your time trial, warm up for 30 minutes on a trainer, rollers, or on the road. During this half hour, slowly ramp up your cadence and resistance until you reach race pace or zone 5. When you begin your race, focus your attention on maintaining your highest level of output. Gradually build your pace until you reach your most effective rpm range. Within a minute of the start, heart-rate levels will consistently go a few beats above your anaerobic threshold. This means you will be working at 90 to 95 percent of your maximum heart rate, something you should have practiced regularly in your training. You may find it helpful to mentally break the time trial into four quarters to make the task less formidable.

As you approach the turnaround or a sharp turn, take a quick drink or give your back a few seconds of relief from the aero posture. You need to slow your bike anyway, so you might as well put this opportunity to good use. Reassume the aero position during the turn and accelerate out of it until you reach your effective rpm zone once again. Try to maintain this cadence until the finish. Numerous studies have shown that when overall power outputs are the same, the riders who ride with consistent speed and power output finish ahead of those who don't.

Mike Sayers, a former long-term pro who was interviewed by the Sacramento Bee before the Amgen Tour of California in 2009, had this to say about racing in time trials: "It basically feels like your head's going to explode. You feel kind of weak. You're going so hard, and your legs have so much blood in them trying to feed those muscles. It feels like you're pedaling squares." Although time trials are uncomfortable, the effort can be well rewarded. The races that mesh in terms of position, power, and endurance are the ones you will remember with pride.

The National Elite Championship held in Carrolton, Kentucky, in 1976 was such a race for me. I had just won the Red Zinger Classic in Colorado the week before and was feeling confident. The advantage of having trained and raced at altitude was apparent. I was riding strong that day, and I remember the excitement I felt as I passed my minute man (starts were separated by one minute) and used the emotional energy generated by the pass to maintain my pace and pass my two-minute man. The pain of the effort was overwhelmed by the exhilaration of my first-place finish, which set a national 25-mile record by nearly two minutes. The pain was nothing compared to that experience!

ROAD RACING

It is my personal feeling that road racing is the essence of cycling. The changes in weather, large distances, speeds that groups can maintain, and the comradery and collaborations involved in a group all characterize this genre of racing. Road racing has been popular throughout the world, especially in Europe, since it became an organized sport in 1868, not long after the advent of the bicycle. The Paris-Roubaix (1868), Tour de France (1903), and Giro d'Italia (1909) remain popular today and have been models for many races all over the world. Road

Masters Cycling Event: El Tour de Tucson

If you like dry, desert air and towering saguaro cacti, this is the event for you. El Tour de Tucson takes place each year in the middle of November in Arizona. The ride supports several charities, including Tu Nidito Children and Family Services, the American Parkinson's Disease Association, Big Brothers and Sisters of Tucson, and the Leukemia and Lymphoma Society. The course is a scenic 109-mile (175 km) loop around the perimeter of Tucson, but shorter routes are available for the less ambitious. El Tour is unique in that it is one of the only events to serve as both a mass-participation ride for all levels of ability and a full-blown road race for elite riders. Although this may seem like a potentially dangerous venue, elite groupings based on racing history and fitness (platinum, gold, and silver) seem to work quite well for getting participants into the correct corrals. El Tour also holds a multiday expo before the event.

El Tour is a good event to ride with a team or with a few fit friends. It is ideal for practicing road-racing skills and strategies and for chasing and bridging the many groups that form at the first river crossing. Two dry riverbed crossings filled with soft, sandy dirt and hard, loose stones require you to dismount and practice your cyclo-cross skills. Serious riders and racers who attend El Tour enjoy the challenge of racing with top-category amateurs and pros. Former winners of the Tour de France have competed in the race: Greg LeMond was honored at the event and Lance Armstrong competed after his hiatus from cycling for cancer treatment.

This event is fun and well organized, and it supports admirable causes. If you are looking for a century-plus ride, this one is well worth your consideration.

races can have mass starts on open or closed roads. For nonelite racers, they may have staggered starts based on classification or age groups. The courses can be flat, rolling, or mountainous. Some are relatively short, and others are held in stages that can span a few weeks. The Milan-San Remo race began in 1907 with a distance of 288 km. Today it approaches 300 km, making it one of the longest single-day races. The Tour de France lasts for 23 days and travels about 3,500 km with some of the stages climbing up the steep mountain roads of the Pyrenees and Alps at grueling paces.

Road racing became a world championship event in 1893, and it has been part of the modern Olympic Games since Athens in 1896. Nearly all road races feature events for masters. USA cycling has had separate national championships for masters cyclists since the 1980s that are staged in five-year age increments. Just as the pros compete for the world title, cyclists can compete against the world's best masters at the UCI World Championships for the ultimate prize, a world championship rainbow jersey.

Preparing to Road Race

Chapter 5 discusses riding on a track as a training tool for other disciplines, and road racing is no exception. Track riding tempers and tunes the muscles, tendons, and ligaments in the legs. It also sharpens the central nervous system to improve neuromuscular response. Some of the best roadies of each era got their starts on the track. Mark Cavendish, Bradley Wiggins, and second-generation star Taylor Phinney started racing on the track, as did five-time Tour de France winner, Eddy Merckx. As a masters cyclist, some of my most successful seasons at the nationals were due to time spent on the track. Ken Fuller, my Olympic teammate, also trains on the track, and he won national road and track championships in the same year.

Track racing requires the continuous recruitment of fast-twitch muscle fibers, thus improving your ability to accelerate quickly (jump) when strategically necessary. No one who saw the final stage of the 2009 Tour de France can forget how George Hincapie, an American, and Mark Renshaw, an Australian, executed a textbook lead-out for Mark Cavendish in the final sprint. Mark Cavendish had a superior jump, shot out from behind Renshaw, and easily held off his competitors to take the stage as Renshaw took second.

Competitive group riding is another way to prepare for road racing, and cycling clubs usually hold organized rides once or twice each week. Identify the stronger riders in the group and work to keep up with them. Scheduled sprints during the ride will test your ability to accelerate quickly and maintain speed until the finish.

Aerodynamics in Road Racing

Chapter 6 covers information about riding in a pack, but additional aerodynamic considerations exist for small groups of racers who want to initiate a breakaway. During a road race, one or more riders may attempt to break away from the main group. Riders who are attempting to escape the field must assume a bent-elbow, low-profile position similar to that of a time-trial racer, but without the aero bars and elbow pads. Without the protection of the peloton, an aerodynamic profile is essential.

Strategies for Road Racing

The main goal of a road racer is to cross the finish line first, and the key to a successful race is to conserve energy. One of the strategies employed to this end is drafting, as chapter 6 discusses. You can join teammates or cooperate with competitors to ride in a pace line or an echelon, which can increase the speed at which you ride and can reduce your energy output by as much as 40 percent. Small groups that attack and break away from the peloton are more likely to succeed than solo breakaways since they can travel faster than the larger group, and the cost in energy to a single rider is so dear. Teams can also work together prevent a breakaway by chasing down the escapees and bringing them back into the main group. They can bring their sprinter to the front of the peloton for a fast finish or assist a member who has punctured a tire in returning to the pack. Doing well in a race is much easier when you have help. Keep in mind that any partnership you form with other competitors will dissolve if one of them cannot maintain pace or as you approach the finish.

Road races vary from 20 to 160 km or more and can take place in one day or over weeks. The strategies will differ accordingly. How you choose to race

Masters Cycling Event: RAGBRAI

The name of this favorite race in the Midwest United States is an acronym for Register's Annual Great Bicycle Ride Across Iowa. It is a billed as a noncompetitive ride across the state. Having said that, I will also tell you that it is nicknamed *The Great Race Across Iowa*, so bragging rights certainly apply. RAGBRAI draws recreational riders from across the United States and abroad. The course travels from the western border to the eastern border of Iowa, stopping in towns across the state. The ride is limited to 8,500 weeklong riders and 1,500 day riders. The length of the route averages 472 miles (760 km). Eight communities are selected each year to host the event, two for the beginning and end points and six for overnight stops en route. The average distance between host communities is 68 miles (110 km). Traditionally, at the beginning of the ride, cyclists dip the rear wheel of their bikes in either the Missouri River or the Big Sioux River, depending on where the ride starts. At the finish, the riders dip their front wheels in the Mississippi River.

The weather during RAGBRAI can be hot since it begins in late July and ends a week later. In 1994, I innocently ventured into the ride, thinking of my days riding and camping at American youth hostels. RAGBRAI turned out to be a weeklong party disguised as a bike ride, a sort of Mardi Gras on bicycles.

depends on your strengths in terms of the competition. The best position in the peloton is in the front third if you want to be a serious competitor. Have faith in your own abilities, and don't let yourself be intimidated by younger riders. Hold that position, especially in a pack of younger rivals who may be more powerful. Use their power to your advantage. As I said in chapter 6, if you are not constantly moving up in the pack, you are probably losing ground to those who are. It is all right to drift back slightly and then move back up, but avoid making jumps to move up, which can sap your energy. Take advantage of broad openings in which you can move up quickly, expending little or no energy on someone else's wheel. As you age, you need to let the stronger riders do your work for you. Let them commit to closing a gap with you on the wheel instead of the other way around.

A common mistake that I see beginners and even some expert masters make is pulling the pack up a hill. This is a terrible position to put yourself in. If you are rolling into a hill with momentum, those behind you will take advantage of the momentum generated by the pack. They may overtake you and drop you off the back. On the other hand, if you are not a strong climber, the best place to be during a longer climb is near the front so that even if you drift back when the inevitable gaps open up, you will still be in the front third of the peloton, rather than dropped off the back. Choose your position and the wheels you sit on with care since an unsteady or inexperienced rider can unintentionally take you down by hitting your front wheel. Riding at the very front consumes a lot of energy, and there is a lot of jockeying for position. Instead, sit a few wheels back in the pack, and let others battle the winds. Take advantage of the strength of others and conserve your energy.

A smart competitor watches other smart competitors from the start, marking them for possible attacks, alliances, and team setups. Learning to recognize the stronger, more-dominant riders is the first step in identifying who can make a break stick and who can't. Avoid riders in the latter category. If a break does go up the road, and you are fortunate enough to be in it, as long as your strength matches that of your partners, do your share of the work and nothing more. Avoid sudden accelerations since they may be perceived as attacks, undermining your alliance.

Watch competitive bicycle races on television for ideas. Jean-Pierre Monseré was a young Belgian rider who won the world professional road championships in Leicester, England in 1970. When asked how he had beaten prerace favorites, Eddy Merckx and Felice Gimondi, he replied that he had watched the amateurs race on the same course the day before on television and had simply mimicked the winning move.

CRITERIUMS AND CIRCUIT RACES

Perhaps the most popular and challenging type of road racing in terms of tactics and experience is the criterium. A number of laps are ridden on short, closed courses that are less than 5K in length, and the race normally takes no more than an hour to complete. Lap primes, or *preems*, are often awarded to the rider who crosses the line on a particular lap first, usually signaled by a bell. The winner of the race is the first rider to cross the finish without being lapped. This kind of cycling event is very popular with spectators since they get to see the riders pass several times during the course of the race.

When I raced in Europe, especially Belgium, criteriums were known as *kermesse*, which is a word for a festival rather than a race. Bicycle races provided the entertainment. They were typically held on short courses, usually no more than one or two city blocks. They were very fast, and in Holland, Belgium, and Germany, they occasionally took place on cobblestones. I remember a points race in Germany with a blazing fast pace right from the gun and 75 men negotiating a tight street course on cobblestones in the rain.

Circuit races are held on longer courses, usually more than 5K per lap, and they often include significant hill climbs to add to the challenge. As with criteriums, circuit races are held on closed courses. The length is determined either by a certain number of laps or a specified time. These races are all about speed, so your preparation should include an aggressive attitude during your training rides. Track racers tend to dominate circuit races, illustrating another benefit of training on the track.

Strategies for Criterium and Circuit Racing

Success in a criterium or circuit race requires a combination of smooth, powerful riding and good technical skill. If you are nervous cornering at high speeds in very close proximity to other riders, avoid crits. They can be unnerving if a rider strikes a pedal during a turn or comes into a turn too hot and falls directly in your line. You will probably go down, taking several others with you like dominoes. Trying to brake and steer around the problem does not work in a pack since you will end up in someone else's line and perhaps cause a worse crash.

If the inherent thrills, dangers, and split-second decisions appeal to you, and you have the technical skills and endurance to sprint repeatedly out of corners, the spunk to aggressively push your way through a crowded field of riders, and the strength to crank out a big gear for the final 500 meters, this is your kind of race. Occasionally, winners emerge from small, well-coordinated breakaways, but the race usually comes down to a final lap sprint. An iron will and pure leg strength will get you to the podium.

CYCLO-CROSS

Cyclo-cross, or CX, is a specialty form of bicycle racing that uses modified road bikes. It usually takes place during the fall and winter. Often described as off-road criteriums, CX consists of laps around a varied course that can include pavement, wooded trails, grass, steep hill climbs and descents, and obstacles that require you to dismount and carry your bike, remounting after you have traversed the obstacles. Masters races typically last an hour or less. They require off-road bike handling skills that can only be acquired with experience.

Preparing for Cyclo-Cross

Cyclo-cross is to mountain bike racing what track racing is to circuit racing. CX requires some serious anaerobic training. For example, your training sessions should include a series of incrementally harder intervals that take you beyond your anaerobic threshold for as long as three minutes. This is accomplished while you ride around a circuit that has turns and obstacles. You will lose speed into the turns and then accelerate out of them, which can be very taxing. Technical skill is also required since you will need to dismount quickly to get over obstacles, carve turns in soft terrain, and perhaps negotiate ankle-deep mud. Try the following series of step-up intervals:

1. Warm up for 15 to 20 minutes in low gears.
2. Ride in a straight line at full speed for 10 seconds to simulate a start.
3. Ride for one minute around a tight circuit that has four left and right turns. Practice jumps out of the saddle to exit the turns.
4. Execute a hard jump at the beginning for three minutes to force yourself past your anaerobic threshold. Next, make a hard, sustained effort that includes four to six turns, a barrier and dismount, and a short, steep hill that requires you to dismount and run.

You and your friends can set up your own circuit off-road that includes any technical features you want to practice. Competing well in CX takes power that is earned by liberal doses of training in zones 4 and 5, endurance obtained from saddle time, and finally, good genes. It's fun and exhilarating, and it brings out the child in most of us. My personal favorite is the Cross-Vegas, an annual race held in conjunction with the world-famous Interbike, a bike show in Las Vegas during October.

Equipment for Cyclo-Cross

CX bikes are lightweight and have drop bars, knobby tires, and cantilever brakes for better clearance in muddy conditions. Unlike the tactical criterium or road race, in which drafting and high speeds are the norm, CX is all about endurance and bike handling skills. A CX racer is permitted to receive mechanical assistance during the race. Racers can have mechanics and pit crews, otherwise known as family and friends, standing by to change out bikes if their machines become gummed up with mud. Bikes are cleaned, lubricated, or repaired before the next lap is completed.

The CX setup generally features a saddle that rides a centimeter or lower than that of a road bike for faster jumps. CX bikes have longer wheelbases and higher bottom brackets for better clearance, and the handlebars may be positioned a bit higher for better maneuvering. You can buy a state-of-the-art CX bike off the shelf, but many CXers are more pragmatic. Instead of trashing brand new equipment or wrecking a new Dura Ace 7900 crankset or derailleur, they prefer to cannibalize components from older bikes that have been gathering dust in the basement or garage. These collections of parts are often mismatched, but when oiled, they work well.

Strategies for Cyclo-Cross

The best approach in cyclo-cross is to get a good start and pace yourself so that you don't blow up early. Try to follow the race leaders as closely as possible so that your participation actually factors in the race, and you will feel good about yourself, regardless of your finish. Try to execute dismounts, stairs, and jumps smoothly, and make every effort to maintain good form and technical efficiency.

MOUNTAIN BIKE (MTB) RIDING AND RACING

Definitely the new kid on the block, MTB racing is more than a hundred years younger than road racing. MTBs were invented in northern California in the 1970s. They received full UCI recognition in 1990 when the first world championships were held in Purgatory, Colorado. The huge popularity of the sport prompted the IOC to include mountain biking in the Summer Olympic Games in Atlanta in 1996.

The National Off-Road Bicycle Association (NORBA) represents MTB racing for USA Cycling and identifies three official categories: endurance, or cross-country, with its roots in CX; downhill or gravity; and ultraendurance. The technically adept can compete in an unofficial category called *trials*, in which daring and incredibly skillful feats are expertly executed, and I can't accurately describe it in words. Footage of these amazing stunts done on mountain bikes and BMX can be viewed on YouTube. Aside from the extreme forms of the sport, mountain bikes give you a way to enjoy the beautiful outdoors away from traffic and the trappings of civilization. If you have never been mountain biking before, you are in for a real treat. You will become reacquainted with your more primitive nature and return home covered with dirt, mud, and perhaps a few scrapes, and you will have fun in the process. You will be able to elevate your bike-handling skills to new levels as you address unexpected obstacles and negotiate difficult terrain.

Preparing for MTB Racing

As with cyclo-cross, adept bike-handling skills and anaerobic workouts are essential if you plan to race. Handling a mountain bike efficiently and skillfully on technical terrain requires a lot of practice, and even the best racers break bones. Consider the interval training from the previous section on cyclo-cross while preparing to race a MTB. High-level conditioning should be directed at your weaknesses, not your strengths. For example, if you are preparing for a technical event and your skills in this area are lacking, train on trails that closely simulate the terrain you will encounter when you race.

Equipment for MTB

Joe Breeze, Gary Fisher, Charlie Cunningham, Keith Bontrager, and Tom Ritchey are often heralded as key figures in the birth of the sport. MTB has come a long way since they modified balloon-tire bikes and beach cruisers to produce machines that were capable of negotiating rough terrain. The mountain bikes that evolved from these early experiments had no suspension, making riding on a rough, jolting trail very uncomfortable. With full suspension, hydraulic-disc brakes, and 27 speeds, today's MTBs bear little resemblance to their predecessors. They are built with features specifically targeting their intended category. They are faster, safer, and more comfortable to ride.

As with every kind of cycling, you should wear a protective helmet and gloves when mountain biking. Off-road trails may require dismounts and hiking, so mountain bike shoes typically have inset tread and cleats. You can use platform pedals without cleats, but you will have more power with the SPD-style clipless pedals you commonly find on mountain bikes. SPD stands for Shimano Pedaling Dynamics, but other pedal system manufacturers make this style of pedal. The bottle cages need to be stronger to keep containers from popping out onto the trail, and you want to be able to adjust your seat height as required.

Positioning on the Bike for MTB

The bike setup for MTB reflects the type of off-road riding you plan to do. If you want to ride on flat, nontechnical fire roads, your position will be similar to that of a road bike with the saddle placed higher to improve leverage on the pedals. If you are on trails that have technical switchbacks, drop-offs, and uneven terrain, place the saddle down to lower your center of gravity. The reach, or stem length, of most cross-country MTBs is less than that of a road bike, and the saddle will be moved back for better traction on steep climbs. MTB cleats are usually adjusted back with the foot forward for better slow-speed torque.

Strategies for MTB

As with CX, masters competitors must be well versed in technical riding skills and possess a great deal of raw courage and endurance. To begin with, forget the racing. Obtain the necessary skills by riding with a MTB group or a friend, and enjoy the satisfaction and natural ambience of being on your bike in the wilderness and feeling the rush of fresh, vegetation-scented air in your face under a blue sky. Take advantage of the suspension to spring over obstacles or catch air in the course of your ride, but always ride with control. I have often felt that the thrill of riding my MTB downhill on a challenging trail is similar to that of downhill skiing without the cost of the lift ticket or the bulky clothing.

The strategy with which you approach racing will be determined by your degree of competitiveness. Less-conditioned riders with good bike-handling skills may be able to compete if they can negotiate difficult terrain smoothly. The main goal is to stay in contact with the race leaders while conserving as much energy as possible. Although this strategy is the hallmark of a strong, competitive effort, it is an advanced approach. Novice racers should focus on observing the moves of experienced racers on specific terrain features. In most races, the field is reduced through attrition, but attacks and counterattacks occasionally occur. When you're just starting to race, take mental notes, and process the information so that you can learn to compete more effectively in future races. Once your conditioning and technique improve, you can attempt the moves yourself.

CENTURIES, DOUBLE CENTURIES, AND BREVETS

Many cyclists, especially serious recreational cyclists, get the urge to push the limits of their endurance by participating in organized long-distance rides. Long-distance rides often wind and climb through scenic surroundings, and they can be relatively flat or mountainous. These events are numerous and can be found all over the world. They range in distance from 100 miles to as many as 1,500 kilometers (about 932 miles). Many races are open to everyone, but some require qualification.

The Century

A century ride is 100 miles (160 km) long. These excursions can be picturesque and a lot of fun. Most rides are supported with rest stops that include beverages and light snacks. Sometimes, local law-enforcement officers stop vehicular traffic at major intersections. Whatever the venue, these rides offer cyclists an opportunity to spend time with friends or make new friends as they pedal their way to the finish.

Preparing to Ride a Century

The more mileage you ride before a century, the better you will feel afterward, but you must increase your mileage gradually. Your goal is to get to the start of the century in the best shape possible and be rested and injury-free. For example, suppose that you can comfortably ride 20 miles (32 km) and your weekly mileage totals around 45 to 50 miles (70-80 km). You will need to allow yourself between two and two and a half months to train, including strength training and stretching. During this time, you will need to increase the distance of your long ride by 5 miles (8 km) each week and your total mileage by 8 to 12 miles (12-20 km) per week until your long ride is about 65 miles (100 km), and your total mileage for the week reaches about 120 miles (193 km). The week before your event, shorten your long ride to 50 miles (80 km) and your total mileage to around 75 (120 km) so that you will be rested for the century. Of

Masters Cycling Event: The Solvang Half and Full Century

The Solvang Century and Half-Century rides begin and end in the town of Solvang (a Norwegian word that means sunny field), a small, quaint Danish community nestled in wooded, rolling hills in the Santa Inez Valley, a few miles north of Santa Barbara, California. The town features true Danish architecture and some of the most pristine country roads imaginable. If you are a cyclist and a connoisseur of wine, Solvang may be the perfect venue for sampling offerings at the local vineyards while pursuing your cycling passion, any time of the year. The organized rides are held in March when wildflowers in full bloom, such as lupine, wild mustard, lilacs, and the golden poppy (California's state flower) add sweeping areas of color to the rolling landscape. The event was started in 1983 by the SCOR Cardiac Cyclists Club of Los Angeles. The money raised supports numerous cycling events and the Make-a-Wish Foundation.

The 100-mile (161 km) ride with an elevation gain of 4,950 feet (1.5 km) loops through the cities of Lompoc, Vandenberg, Santa Maria, and Los Olivos before heading back to Solvang. The 50-mile (80 km) route loops out to Lompoc and back, and the first 23 miles (37 km) follow the same route as the century. The total elevation gain of the half century is 1,850 feet (564 m), and no hill on either course is taller than 800 feet (244 m).

Solvang also boasts a double century for ultradistance cyclists and the insanely ambitious. The ride covers 193 actual miles (310 km) as it heads through the beautiful Santa Inez Valley up to Morrow Bay and back through San Luis Obispo, Pismo Beach, and Los Alamos. The total elevation gain is around 7,500 feet (2.3 km). This ride is one of a number of double-century rides all over the state of California that are scheduled between February and November. Finishing any three of them will garner you the triple crown.

course, cyclists who are used to cranking out more miles can prepare in less time or train to ride a faster century.

Strategies for a Century

A ride of this distance may seem formidable to some, but even inexperienced long-distance cyclists can get to the finish if they pace themselves. This is not a sprint. If you are new to long-distance cycling, ride easily, take breaks, and eat frequently to prevent your blood sugar from dropping too low. Once you have bonked, it's difficult to recover, and the remainder of your ride could be torturous. Staying hydrated will also help you to maintain energy, so be sure to refill your bottles at rest stops. If you have ridden for hours without peeing, you're not drinking enough. Enjoy your ride! When you reach the finish, your legs may be tired and your backside may be tender, but you will have accomplished something that most people haven't. You will have covered 100 miles under your own power!

The Double Century

Double centuries, as you might expect, are 200 miles (320 km) long, and if you're thinking about doing one, I'm assuming that you have several or more centuries under your belt and are looking for new challenges. Riding a double century is definitely that: a challenge. It will take you to degrees of fatigue you have never felt before, and it will test your resolve to finish.

Preparing for a Double Century

As you are likely to spend at least 12 hours in the saddle, a good bike fit and a bike that is in good working order is essential. You will want to carry two or three large water bottles and packets of powdered energy drinks to mix with the water. Your ride will likely start or end in the dark, so you will need a light, and you should wear reflective clothing. Carry a windbreaker and arm and leg warmers for when it becomes cool. You will be expending a lot of calories, and you may become easily chilled later in the ride. Carry tools for emergency repairs, including a chain breaker, Allen wrenches, tire irons, small screw driver, and a spoke wrench. You will also want to carry a couple of spare tubes, CO_2 cartridges, patch kit, and a spare tire in case one is damaged beyond repair. This may sound like a lot of stuff to carry, but you don't want to be stuck out in the middle of nowhere with no help in sight.

Increase your mileage gradually, and ride four or five days per week, doing easy recovery rides after long, fast rides. For example, if you average around 90 to 100 miles (145-160 km) per week, and you can comfortably ride 50 miles, it will probably take you about three to four months to train for a 200-mile ride. You should do one to two long rides and two to three shorter rides per week. If you do two long rides of 60 to 80 miles (100-130 km) on Saturday and Sunday, then Monday's ride will be a short, easy recovery spin. You should set one day per week aside for rest from any form of exercise except for stretching. Unlike century training, you will not steadily increase your mileage. Instead, you will train in waves, allowing your total weekly mileage to drop periodically for recovery. You may want to include fast century rides as part of your training, or even back-to-back centuries a couple of weeks before your event to test your fitness.

Strategies for a Double Century

Stretch your body thoroughly to warm up, and stay off the bike until the start. You can warm up on the bike during the beginning of the 200 miles ahead of you. You should have determined what works for you nutritionally during your training. Don't try anything new during your ride since you want to minimize your risk for nausea or intestinal disturbances for the 11 to 14 hours you may be on the road. You should be prepared to consume about 300 calories per hour and have an emergency supply of energy bars and gels to keep you from bonking between rest stops. Stay hydrated.

You will need to pace yourself throughout the ride, especially if the terrain is hilly. Shift your position on the bike frequently to give your muscles, spine, and backside some relief. Stretch thoroughly when you stop to snack and refill your bottles. This is a test of endurance and resolve, so ride one mile at a time and don't think too far ahead. It may help to mount or wear a GPS unit so that you can monitor your progress along the route. You may be exhausted and sore at the end of the ride, but give yourself a well-deserved pat on the back for a wonderful achievement!

The Brevet

Brevets, or *randonnées* (long rambles in the countryside), are unsupported, ultradistance cycling events that can range from 200K (124 miles) to 1500K (932 miles). These rides for endurance cyclists can be found all over the world. Since no outside support is provided, participants, or *randonneurs*, must be self-sufficient. They are permitted to buy necessary supplies along the route. However, vehicular support is not permitted, except at checkpoints. Preparation and strategies for these events are similar to that for a double century. The amount of base mileage depends on the length of the brevet. Qualification

Masters Cycling Event: The Paris-Brest-Paris Brevet

The inaugural Paris-Brest-Paris (PBP) Brevet was held in 1891 and was a race for professional cyclists. However, it is now a timed, noncompetitive ride for amateur endurance cyclists. This 1200K from Paris to the coastal town of Brest and back is held once every four years. Every participant must first qualify by completing a series of brevets during the same year. For qualification, *randonneurs*, or riders, must complete brevets of 200K (125 miles), 300K (190miles), 400K (250 miles), and 600K (370 miles) within the specified time limits.

Riders must finish within 84 or 90 hours, depending on their group. Fifteen checkpoints are spread out along the route, and the distances between them range from 53 to 85 miles (85-137 km). Only some of the checkpoints have food, so self-sufficiency is imperative. Vehicular support is forbidden on the course. For $45 USD, riders can pick up bags of food and drink at two designated points along the route. Since the clock is always running, riders grab a few hours of sleep in a dorm room, on a gymnasium floor, or even on a park bench when they are too tired to go on. Front and rear lights (with extra bulbs) and reflective gear are required for night riding. Participants must also carry food, extra beverages, gear for foul weather, and tools for any necessary repairs; consequently, they mount bags on their bikes to accommodate these necessities.

If you think this event sounds grueling, you are right. Still, surviving a ride like this is something you will never forget. Every finisher receives a commemorative medal to document the achievement. One finisher put it like this, "This is a major happening, not just a bike ride. It's not as hard as you might think, and it's definitely worth doing at least once."

rides may be necessary for the longer brevets, such as the Paris-Brest-Paris. Time limits for completing the events range from 13.5 hours for the 200K to 116.4 hours for the 1400K distance.

Whether you are a competitive racer, an endurance animal, a serious recreational cyclist, or a weekend warrior, a variety of races and rides exist to accommodate cyclists of all abilities and types. Organized events give you the opportunity to socialize, improve your cycling skills, and test your level of fitness. You will take away lasting memories of your experiences.

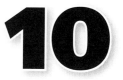

Dealing With Injuries and Setbacks

It's difficult to come away from hours and hours in the saddle completely unscathed. You can try to prepare yourself for hard training by stretching and strengthening your body, but sometimes you need to do some tweaking to find out what really works for your individual idiosyncrasies. Try adding variety to your training program by changing your routes and the time of the day that you head out on rides. This will both reduce your risk for overuse injuries and help prevent burnout. Regardless of the efforts you make to avoid them, issues can arise that are annoying and sometimes painful.

SADDLE SORES

You may have experienced discomfort in the saddle when you first started to ride seriously. A bicycle saddle is designed to support the body, placing most of the pressure on the ischial tuberosities, or sit bones. Pain or discomfort in this area is a very common complaint, which is due to an improper bike setup or mainly from cyclists who have not yet logged many hours on the road. As you gradually add mileage in the saddle, the soft tissue covering your sit bones will become tougher, and this discomfort will eventually fade.

A far more annoying affliction is the saddle sore, which develops from repeated and extended abrasion of the skin on the perineum and the lower buttocks, which are under pressure when the pedals are pumped. Moisture and heat from perspiration add to the friction and exacerbate trauma to the tissue. The area may become red and inflamed. Cyclists who log hundreds of miles per week may experience skin ulcers, which are craterlike in appearance. Minor saddle sores can become very painful and inflamed if they become infected. Infection may occur in hair follicles, causing furuncles, or small boils, to develop. These boils initially feel like small pimples, but they many grow into larger, painful, puss-filled lumps if you do not take care of them.

The chamois in the seat of bicycle shorts harbors bacteria that cannot be destroyed using normal laundering techniques without ruining your shorts. People differ in their sensitivity to infection, so you must choose the plan that best keeps your bum healthy. The best course of action is preventive. A number of products, such as stick lubricants, medicated petroleum jelly, or lubricating gels and creams, can be applied to sensitive areas to prevent abrasions. My personal favorite is a product that was developed by athletes for athletes. Okole Stuff is a chamois ointment that contains lanolin, allantoin, tea-tree oil, and aloe.

In addition to lubricating them, make sure your cycling shorts fit comfortably and have adequate padding. Spraying the chamois of your shorts with Lysol or another disinfectant before laundering will kill the bacteria that normal washings will not. As previously mentioned in chapter 9, cycling shorts are designed to be worn commando. The seams and edges of undergarments will cause painful chafing, especially if you are accumulating a lot of mileage.

You should also find yourself an anatomically friendly saddle. This may require some experimentation in terms of shape and design. Many bike stores will allow you to return a saddle if it doesn't work for you. You can reduce

Feminine Cycling Issues

For many years, women were forced to ride on bicycle seats that were not designed for their anatomy. Chafing, inflammation, and even genital irritation and swelling followed hours in the saddle, making urination or showering after a long ride extremely painful. Terry was the first company to come out with a saddle that gave women some relief. Today, women can choose from several female-friendly saddles that aren't necessarily more expensive. Cheaper saddles may break down sooner, but if they fit your body better, you can afford to replace them more often.

Even with equipment modification, problems can still occur for women who put in a lot of miles. If you experience genital swelling, icing the area may give you some relief. If the swelling is firm, red, and hot to the touch, you may have an infection that requires antibiotics. See your general practitioner or gynecologist. Women can also get the same pressure ulcers and abscesses that men get. If you tend to get vaginal infections, take off your cycling shorts as soon as possible after your ride, and spray the chamois with a disinfectant, such as Lysol, before laundering.

friction by making sure your saddle is adjusted correctly. Pedaling should not result in excessive bobbing and shifting from side to side. While training for the RAAM, my mileage peaked between 550 and 600 miles (885-965 km) each week, and I found that I got the most relief from changing saddles or bikes every few days. The subtle differences in the width and shape of the saddle changed the location of my pressure points just enough to prevent sores from forming.

Some masters cyclists dislike the traditional horned saddle. I have found it causes me to lose feeling in my lower back when I put in a lot of miles. The horseshoe-shaped Adamo saddle by ISM is an alternative to consider. The horseshoe is open in the front. Adjusting the tilt and the fore and aft positioning is critical to its use, but I have found this saddle to be the most comfortable of any I have yet tried.

ROAD RASH

Those who ride say that there are two kinds of cyclists: those who have crashed and those who are going to crash. Eventually all cyclists will deal with road rash, or the flaying of flesh by asphalt, concrete, or dirt. Ouch! Depending on the severity, road rash can be very painful during the healing process. It can cover a relatively large area of skin, making the wound difficult to bandage, which creates risk of infection. It usually occurs on an area that will come into painful (and sometimes messy) contact with clothing or bed sheets.

First, if you are not too damaged, get back on your bicycle and go home before the inevitable stiffness sets in. Air on the wound will initially sting, but the discomfort will soon fade. When you reach home, thoroughly clean the site with mild soap or irrigate it with a wash bottle of a sterile 0.9 percent solution of sodium chloride (table salt). This will remove any foreign matter. If necessary, use sterile gauze and gently swab the area to remove any lingering debris. Some physicians advise bathing the area with hydrogen peroxide, but there are data that suggest this practice may further damage the tissue, impeding healing. Do not scrub the area too aggressively since this could also cause additional tissue damage. When the wound is completely clean, apply an antibiotic ointment and fix a sterile dressing to the area with adhesive tape. Change the dressing at least every few days, and keep the area moist with ointment and a bandage until it is healed. This aids the healing process by promoting healthy tissue formation to minimize scarring and prevent infection.

Road rash is the primary reason why serious cyclists shave their legs. It's true that a sharp-looking kit looks less professional on a man with hairy legs, and the bike-fashion police might haul you off in irons if you don't shave, but the real reason for shaving is far more practical. Hairless legs are easier to clean and bandage, and the absence of hair reduces the opportunity for infection. Triathletes also have a hydrodynamic advantage; however, the aerodynamic advantage for cyclists is negligible. Shaved legs do have some disadvantages. They must be continually maintained to prevent stubble and ingrown hairs. An alternative to shaving is waxing, but I haven't known too many men that would even try that painful ritual once, let alone repeat it. Women who wax are tough!

Hillard Salas

I met Hill Salas and his wife, Angie, three years ago after the Las Vegas Marathon. Hill had finished his first marathon, and he looked very fit. I also learned that he is an avid cyclist and couldn't decide whether he was a cyclist who runs or a runner who rides a bike.

Hill started cycling in 1986, inspired by Greg LeMond, who won his first Tour de France that year. He had finished his first year at Michigan State University and had gained the dreaded freshmen fifteen. He rode recreationally, and after getting a job in one of the research labs at the university, one of the professors invited him to join his cycling group. Hill bought a better bike and began to challenge himself with speed and distance.

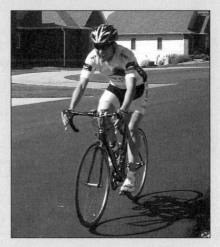

Hill Salas starting out on a training ride.

After finishing college and moving on to medical school at the University of Iowa, he joined the Bicyclists of Iowa City and did tours around the area. He rode on some of the weekend rides and practiced on a trainer when the weather wouldn't permit outdoor cycling.

That summer, Hill raced as a citizen in the Old Capitol Criterium in Iowa City. He finished in the top six each of the five times he did the race with one win and a second-place finish. He rode RAGBRAI once before he met and married Angie. "I managed to find a rider who rode at about the same pace and had a similar philosophy: start early, ride the miles, and get to the campground before the masses to grab a shower. I was mostly with the non-party crowds since I was off and riding at dawn. Overall, I had a great time."

After obtaining a faculty position, he had considerably more demands on his time, especially since he and his wife had two children by this time. Private practice placed severe time constraints on him, and the area where he and his family were living was not ideal for cycling. A couple of years later, he relocated to Dubuque, which turned out to be a good move for him professionally and personally since he could get out on his bike more frequently. "One fall day, I was out riding across town on one of my favorite routes, when a pickup truck, going in the opposite direction, made a left turn right into me, sending me to the pavement on my shoulder. I had a broken collarbone, a scraped shin, and a cracked helmet, and I was off the bike for a couple of months."

After Hill started riding again, his wife Angie challenged him to a 5K running race in Las Vegas that December. "I trained on the treadmill Angie runs on during the winter months. When I finished the race, I thought I had done pretty well, but then some 10-year-old passed me near the finish as if I were standing still! I saw the picture of Angie and me after the race and didn't recognize myself; I thought I was looking at the Michelin Man! A look at the scale gave me some bad news; I weighed 180 pounds (81 kg), 30 pounds (14 kg) heavier than better days."

For Hill, this was the motivation he needed to begin a fitness and performance regimen. He continued to run to get into better shape for cycling, joined a local bike club with speedy members, and went on the club's Wednesday rides. He raced in a 10K run in 2005 that Angie had suggested and was nearly fast enough for an age-group medal. He also did a local time trial and placed fourth in the untimed bike division. He decided to try the state road-race championships, and although he didn't place, he did well enough to continue cycling. Since then, Hill has placed in a number of cycling and running events in the age-group category and got an age-group win in a half marathon. He qualified for the Boston Marathon and ran it twice. "At 42, I'm in the best shape of my life; I have better endurance and better sport-specific strength. As a physician, I still have demands on my time, but I can do four to six events in a year. I want to win our local time trial and have another go at the state road championships, winning this time!"

BROKEN COLLARBONES

Lance Armstrong shattered his collarbone in a crash that landed him in a ditch during a five-stage race in Spain in March of 2009. George Hincapie broke his collarbone in a crash in the 17th stage of the Tour de France that same year. Armstrong ended up with a titanium plate bolted into his clavicle and was able to race in the Giro d'Italia in May. Hincapie finished the Tour with his injury, sometimes riding on cobblestones. It was the first time Armstrong had broken his collarbone in his 17 years as a pro. My collarbones remained intact for my first 25 years of road racing and criteriums. At the age of 38, I started racing mountain bikes in the masters category. Within three years, I had collected three broken collarbones from crashes. Now I have built-in coat hooks between my shoulders.

Broken collarbones are common following bicycle crashes; if several riders go down, one may break a clavicle while the rest escape with various degrees of road rash. It's the luck of the fall, so to speak. Elite cyclists are at a higher risk because they typically have very little upper-body musculature, providing less protection for a bone that is already close to the surface of the skin. Collarbone fractures often occur when the rider tries to break his or her fall with an extended arm, which applies excessive force to the clavicle. Hanging onto the handlebars and riding down with the bike will minimize the opportunity for fractures. This technique can be practiced with slow crashes on soft grass. Fortunately, collarbones heal quickly with or without surgery. Getting surgery to pin the collarbone into place yields better cosmetic results and gets you back on the bike more quickly. While the bone is healing, you can spend time on the trainer to stay in shape, but point the handlebars up and keep your body in an upright position. Avoid any jarring motions that could cause movement along the fracture site, impeding the healing process.

Make sure you are receiving all-around good nutrition and getting your daily requirement of calcium, which will facilitate your recovery. Data have shown that external devices, such as ultrasound, electrical stimulation, and magnets, do not accelerate the mending of fractures unless you have a medical condition that inhibits the natural healing process.

KNEE PAIN

The most frequent complaint I hear from masters cyclists who come to me for corrective fitting is about knee pain. The knees are the largest joints in the body and do the lion's share of the work; therefore, they suffer the majority of joint injuries. Many consider cycling to be an activity that spares the knees because of its low-impact nature, but the repetitive motion of pedaling, especially under a load, can lead to a number of overuse injuries. The pain results not from severe inflammation of the soft tissue but from chronic degeneration.

Cyclists in every tier of expertise are at risk for debilitating knee injuries. Sudden increases in mileage or intensity and biomechanical discrepancies can generate a variety of knee-related issues, such as patellar (kneecap) pain, iliotibial band syndrome, and ligament strains. When diagnosing the source of knee pain, you must consider inflexibility, imbalances in muscular strength, misalignment of the kneecap and femur, and discrepancies in leg length, whether congenital or acquired. All of these contributing factors can be corrected, but your bicycle and its geometry relative to your anatomy are critical components.

Knees are less prone to injury if the supporting muscles are strong. Single-leg balancing exercises are excellent for increasing stability. First, try standing on one leg while moving the free leg forward, to the side, and to the back for 10 cycles on each leg. Repeat the cycle twice. When you become comfortable with that routine, add a balance board or a bosu ball to intensify the exercise. Many yoga postures are balance-oriented and help strengthen your stabilizing muscles.

In spite of our best efforts to minimize knee injuries, aging exacts a certain amount of wear and tear on our joints. Studies have shown that the synovial fluid that lubricates the joints loses viscosity as we age. Currently, products are available that have demonstrated efficacy in maintaining joint health, such as the generic compounds glucosamine, chondroitin (a glycosaminoglycan), and methylsulfonylmethane (MSM). Another important compound is hyaluronan, a polysaccharide of high molecular weight that is also a member of the glycosaminoglycan (GAG) family of compounds. It is present in the epithelial, connective, and neural tissues, and it increases the synovial fluid's viscosity and keeps cartilage moist and resilient. Hyaluronan has been used by medical professionals to treat osteoarthritis of the knee, and products containing the compound, such as Runovia, have become popular supplements for athletes, especially runners.

Another product that deserves mention is Omega 3L from Great HealthWorks, which contains essential omega-3 fatty acids extracted from the oil of the species *perna canaliculus* (the green-lipped mussel from New Zealand), one of which is a GAG. It does not contain any shellfish proteins, so it is tolerable for people with allergies.

In spite of the effort we make to keep our bodies healthy and functioning efficiently, sometimes we suffer knee pain. Injuries can occur, and tearing occurs either in the ligaments that attach the muscles to the bones or in the cartilage forming the meniscus, causing debilitating pain. Surgery may be required to repair the damage and restore function. These types of injuries can cause serious interruptions in an athlete's training program.

Osteoarthritis

No matter how carefully we train or adjust our equipment, aging takes its toll on joints and cartilage, especially in the hips and knees. More than 20,000,000 people in the United States alone have debilitating joint pain. Osteoarthritis, often known as wear-and-tear arthritis, occurs as the cartilage simply wears away. It is the most common form of arthritis and the most common reason for replacement surgeries of the hips and knees. Current diagnostic methods cannot detect osteoarthritis until the disease is advanced; however, in a modified approach currently under evaluation, MRI (magnetic resonance imaging) is used to detect the concentration of GAG, which is recognized as a biomarker for osteoarthritis and degenerative-disc disease. A low concentration of GAG in the cartilage indicates the onset of osteoarthritis. Early detection can allow for drug or supplement therapy, potentially preventing surgery in the future.

Acetaminophen (Tylenol) and nonsteroidal anti-inflammatory drugs (NSAIDs), such as Motrin, Advil, and Aleve, have been effective in relieving the joint pain associated with osteoarthritis. These drugs are usually the first course of action in treatment. However, many athletes have found that taking a combination of glucosamine, chondroitin sulfate, and MSM helps relieve knee pain. These compounds provide the natural materials for joint maintenance that our bodies no longer make in sufficient quantities as we age. Glucosamine is an amino sugar that the body distributes in cartilage and other connective tissue. Chondroitin sulfate is a complex carbohydrate that helps cartilage retain water. Methylsulfonylmethane (MSM) is another nutrient essential for joints, cartilage, hair, teeth, and nails. Much of the positive information on this regimen is anecdotal, and the results from current double-blind clinical studies are conflicting. Some people find relief from this regimen and others do not. Personally, I think it's worth a try as an alternative to drug therapy, which can have side effects, or knee-replacement surgery, which can involve considerable downtime.

Chondromalacia

Chondromalacia patellae, or patellofemoral pain syndrome (PFPS), occurs when the cartilage that lines the patella (kneecap) becomes irritated. Normally, this cartilage glides over the joint when the knee is bent, but a strength imbalance between the medial and lateral muscles of the quadriceps can cause the kneecap to track incorrectly and rub against one side of the joint. Weakness in the vastus medialis oblique (VMO) muscle can also contribute to PFPS. Of the four quadriceps muscles, three pull the patella laterally (to the outside). Only the VMO pulls the kneecap medially (to the inside).

An improper bike fit or cleat position can contribute to chondromalacia. Women are more vulnerable to chondromalacia because the angle between their hips and knees is wider than men's. This is sometimes called the *Q-angle*, or the measurement of the angle formed by the intersection of a vertical line through the kneecap and a line from the hip to the kneecap. You can use ibuprofen or naproxen for pain during rehabilitation, which should focus on getting the kneecap to track in a straight line during extension and flexion of the quadriceps. You can change your tracking patterns by balancing your strength evenly among the quadriceps muscles, strengthening the VMO, and making sure your bike position and cleats are properly adjusted.

Cruciate and Collateral Ligament Injuries

The cruciate ligaments are about 2 inches (5 cm) long and give the knees their posterior and anterior stability. The ACL (anterior cruciate ligament) and PCL (posterior cruciate ligament) are located inside the joint capsule and the synovial membrane. The medial collateral ligament (MCL) is outside of the joint on the inner edge of the knee and attaches to the fibula (small bone in the lower leg) and the femur (upper-leg bone). The lateral collateral ligament (LCL) is located outside of the joint on the outer edge of the knee and is attached to the tibia (large bone in the lower leg) and the femur. Injuries to knee ligaments occur when the knee joint is bent and then twisted. This type of injury can happen to overly ambitious cyclists, runners, skiers, or those who engage in contact sports in which ligament strains or tears are common.

Cycling for Life

Jim Penseyres

Jim Penseyres began riding a bike recreationally with his wife in the early 1970s. A decade later, he began cycling to work, and a few more years later, he was competing in USCF (United States Cycling Federation) races. Jim has finished three solo RAAMs, improving his time with each race, and has ridden as part of four-man and eight-man teams with his brother, Pete. In 1989, RAAM included a Human-Powered Vehicle (HPV) division for the first time in its history. Jim and Pete, along with two other cyclists holding impressive credentials (Bobby Fourney and Michael Coles), rode the 2,908 miles (4,700 km) from Costa Mesa, California, to New York City in a two-wheeled recumbent with nose cones on the front and rear of the vehicle and an adjustable Lycra skin. Riding in shifts, they reached the finish line in five days, one hour, and eight minutes, a RAAM average-speed record that holds today at 24.02 miles per hour (39 kph).

The most amazing thing about Jim's considerable cycling accomplishments is that he did it all as an amputee. During the Vietnam War, Jim was assigned to the second battalion in the third Marine division and was on patrol outside of Da Nang. "We were a reaction force," Jim told me, "that was used when other units were in trouble. While on patrol, I stepped on a land mine that removed my leg below the left knee and a section of my right calf. I received two Purple Hearts during my tour, and that was the second."

Jim spent six months in the Oakland Naval Hospital recovering from his

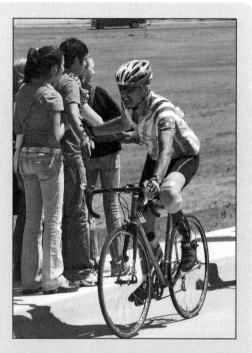

Jim Penseyres on a Ride 2 Recovery tour.

wounds. For rehabilitation, Jim began to surf again. Although surfing was enjoyable and comforting, Pete's successful exploits in ultradistance cycling attracted Jim to the sport of endurance cycling. Jim joined the CAF's (Challenged Athletes Foundation) Operation Rebound in 2008. He mentors many veterans who want to become active again after being seriously injured during military service.

Another organization that Jim passionately supports is the Wounded Warriors: Ride 2 Recovery Project. "What a great program John Wordin has set up!" Jim says with enthusiasm. "I've been waiting 40 years for something like this to come along. Ride 2 Recovery takes men and women who have been wounded mentally or physically while serving our country in the armed forces and introduces them to the world of cycling. They are given bicycles that they can keep, and John sets up several 300- to 450-mile (480-720 km) rides over multiple days with other veterans. During the rides, we pass by many schools, and young children line the streets and wave American flags while shouting words of encouragement. The healing process that this program supports for our wounded warriors is so far reaching that we may never know the full extent of its success."

Jim has had the opportunity to speak in depth with the people involved in the program and has listened to their concerns and frustrations about how their present circumstances will affect their future lives. Jim, speaking from his own experiences, shared this gem of wisdom with those veterans: "Life may not seem fair; that is true, but what you do with what you have left will determine your success in life. One needs to look at these injuries as inconveniences, not disabilities."

Torn ACLs are difficult to heal without surgical repair because when the tear occurs, the site is bathed in synovial fluid, preventing blood from surrounding the wound. Without blood, healing cannot occur. A torn ACL alters the mechanical function of the knee, causing it to lose stability. The ligament may experience microtearing, which doesn't require surgery, a partial rupture, which may or may not require surgery, or a complete rupture, which must be surgically repaired if you plan to do anything that puts lateral pressure on the knee.

PCL injuries result from the application of a great deal of force to the knee when it is bent, such as when a knee sharply hits the dashboard of a car during an accident. Although they are uncommon, they are more frequently experienced by American football players. These injuries, which mostly consist of partial tears, have the potential to heal on their own. For cyclists, MCLs are the knee ligament most commonly hurt.

Injuries can occur when mileage and intensity are increased too quickly. You may feel a pop at the time of the injury. Pain and swelling are common symptoms. You should see a sports physician to determine the extent of the damage. Suggested treatment may include applying ice to reduce the swelling and wearing a brace to stabilize the knee. Exercises should be done during the rehabilitation period, including stationary cycling and drills that strengthen the quadriceps, the muscles that support the knees. Depending on its extent, the injury may take between two and four weeks to heal. Once you're back in the saddle, you should initially ride in lower gears at a high rpm. Increase your mileage by no more than 10 percent per week. Avoid pushing big gears too soon, or you may reinjure the ligament.

Meniscus Tears

The lateral and medial menisci consist of tough cartilage and are responsible for distributing your body weight evenly across the knee and for increasing the stability of the joint. Do not confuse them with the articular cartilage that caps the ends of the bones. If the load on the knee is unbalanced, excessive force is applied to areas of the bone, which can cause excessive wear to the articular cartilage and lead to early osteoarthritis. The meniscus sits between the articular-cartilage caps on the femur and the tibia, or shinbone. Its wedged shape prevents the rounded end of the femur from sliding off the tibia, increasing the stability of the joint.

Menisci rip for the same reasons that ligaments are injured. Symptoms include knee pain, swelling, tenderness of the meniscus under pressure, a clicking sound in the knee, and a decreased range of motion. MRIs are required to see the extent of the injury, and treatment depends on the type of tear. If the tear causes discomfort when the knee is used, a common treatment is to trim the torn part of the meniscus through arthroscopic surgery. Following repair, most people can resume walking the week after the surgery, running within a month, and sports in four to eight weeks.

NECK, SHOULDER, AND BACK PAIN

Neck, shoulder, and back pain are common among cyclists and are influenced by riding posture and technique. They can usually be traced to poor conditioning, inflexibility, or a poorly fit bike. A strong core, regular stretching, and a proper bike fitting will minimize these issues. Some yoga postures specifically target the spine, stretching it and twisting it to increase your range of motion. When stress is applied in these areas, a number of issues can begin to plague you, especially if you spend long hours in the saddle. Each of these problems can be addressed using adjustments that help reduce the amount of stress being applied to specific areas.

Hyperextension

Riding with your hands in the drops for long periods hyperextends the neck and strains the arms, shoulders, and upper back. This can result in painful back spasms if the stress is not relieved. Not counting the helmet, the average human head weighs between 4.5 and 5 kilograms (about 10 pounds). This explains the source of stress on the neck. Aero bars that are too long can exacerbate the problem. Increasing the height of the handlebars or using smaller drops may help reduce the stress. If your top tube is too long, you can compensate by using a shorter stem. Make sure your elbows are soft (not locked), and change your hand position frequently, moving from the tops to the drops to the brake hoods.

Lower-Back Pain

Posture on the bike is also critical. Handlebars that are positioned too low or a top tube stem combination that is too short cause your spine to curve in an exaggerated concave fashion, increasing pressure on the lower back. An overly forward-tilting pelvis usually results in tight quadriceps and can also strain the lower back.

SKIN DAMAGE

With an average surface area of more than 19 square feet (6 square m) and a weight of more than 24 pounds (11 kg), your skin represents the body's largest organ. It performs many remarkable functions. It makes you more attractive to look at by covering the details of your organs, musculature, and skeletal structure and giving you shape. It helps regulate your body temperature by providing surface area for the evaporation of perspiration through the pores and glands. It contains sebaceous (oil) glands to keep itself moist and a combination of nerve endings and fine hairs that give you the sensations of touching and feeling. Vitamin D, which is necessary for protection against infection and cell repair, is manufactured in the skin. This synthesis is catalyzed by exposure to sunlight.

Our skin is subject to a lot of abuse during cycling or other outdoor activities. One such abuse with the potential for long-term consequences is sun exposure. From the time that I began to ride seriously throughout most of my competitive years as an elite cyclist, only two substances were available for protection from the sun: sun-tanning lotion and zinc oxide. The promise made by Coppertone, a popular tanning lotion, of "a magnificently deep, fast tan" gives you an idea of what people thought of sun exposure at the time. I wore Coppertone lotion on my body during bike rides and zinc oxide on my nose while lifeguarding. These practices did little to protect my fair skin from sun damage, although my nose was in good shape. Permanent damage to the skin can occur by as early as age 18 in people who have had frequent exposure to the sun.

Visible light is only a very small segment of the electromagnetic spectrum, which includes low-energy radio waves at one end and high-energy gamma rays at the other end. Ultraviolet (UV) radiation is invisible to the eye and has shorter waves; therefore, it is more energetic than visible light. It damages collagen fibers, thus accelerating aging of the skin. UV rays were divided into three categories when the medical profession began using the radiation for therapeutic reasons. UVA consists of longer-wave (lower-energy) ultraviolet light, which is emitted at wavelengths between 400 and 315 nanometers. UVB is emitted at wavelengths 315 to 280 nanometers, and UVC emits at less than 280 nanometers. The shorter the wavelength, the more energetic and potentially damaging it is. Nearly 99 percent of the UV radiation reaching the earth's surface is UVA.

The intensity of UVA changes little, regardless of the time of day or the season. It penetrates the skin's epidermis and dermis to reach the subcutaneous tissue, causing the skin to age prematurely. It can also penetrate the glass in car windshields. Because UVA does not cause the skin to burn, its sun-protection factor (SPF) cannot be measured. Once thought to be relatively safe, UVA has been shown to cause indirect DNA damage by generating free radicals and reactive oxygen species; hence, it contributes to skin cancer.

UVB causes direct structural damage to cellular DNA. The intensity is highest between 10 a.m. and 2 p.m. and is higher in the summer than in the winter months. It cannot penetrate glass or plastic. However, it can penetrate the epidermis and the dermal skin layer and is the wavelength range responsible for tanning and sunburns. UVA and UVB destroy vitamin A in the skin, which may inflict additional damage. Skin cells that are damaged by UVB do not manufacture sufficient amounts of hyaluronan, causing the skin to age more rapidly.

UVC is almost completely absorbed by the ozone layer and is not a concern in most places on the planet. In the last 50 years, chemicals have been released into the air, reacting in the presence of sunlight with the ozone in the Antarctic. This causes a large hole in this protective layer to open every spring and close again in midsummer. Consequently, the amount of UVC that reaches southern Australia has increased dramatically, and this country has the highest incidence of skin cancer in the world. UVC is completely absorbed in the epidermal layer. With regulations restricting the use of ozone-damaging chemicals, such as chlorofluorocarbons (CFCs), the hole in the ozone layer is very slowly being repaired. However, it will be decades before the ozone resumes its condition of 50 years ago.

Unless you live in southern Australia, broad-spectrum sunscreens that protect against UVA and UVB exposure are sufficient. Use them generously before riding your bike, and be sure to reapply if you are perspiring a great deal. If you live in an area where UVC is an issue, you must use lotions or creams that contain zinc oxide or titanium dioxide to block all wavelengths of UV radiation. Lotions are now available that disperse these pigments colloidally (in very small particles) so that they are transparent and not opaque like the ointments of old. You can

Prevention Is Better Than a Cure

When skin cells are exposed to excessive UV radiation, the structure of their DNA is damaged, and they cannot function correctly. The affected cells must repair themselves before they can replicate. If the cells are too damaged, one or more of the following conditions may occur: irreversible dormancy, apoptosis (cell suicide), or unregulated cell division, which can become cancer. The three types of skin cancer are as follows:

Basal Cell Carcinoma

This carcinoma accounts for 90 percent of all skin cancers in the United States. It appears as small, fleshy nodules on the head, neck, or hands. People at the greatest risk are Caucasians with light hair, eyes, and complexions. The cure rate is 95 percent.

Squamous Cell Carcinoma

This carcinoma may appear either as nodules or as red, scaly patches of skin. It is found on the edges of the ear, face, lips, and mouth. It can spread to other parts of the body. Again, fair-skinned Caucasians are at the greatest risk for this type of cancer. The American Academy of Dermatology reports that 200,000 people are diagnosed with this type of skin cancer each year. Although it is more aggressive than basal cell carcinoma, the cure rate is 95 percent.

Malignant Melanoma

This type of cancer cell is found in the melanocytes, or the cells that produce the pigment melanin, which causes the skin to tan. This rare form accounts for 75 percent of all deaths from skin cancer. Symptoms include changes in the size, shape, or color of a mole; oozing or bleeding from a mole; or the presence of a mole that feels itchy, hard, lumpy, swollen, or sore. Malignant melanoma can spread to other parts of the body through the lymph system or the blood stream. Although fair-skinned people are at higher risk, people with other skin types can also be affected. Early diagnosis is essential for successful treatment.

Having had many basal cell carcinomas removed from my face, hands, and head, I have paid a painful price for the lack of information available about sun exposure before the 1990s. Early sunscreens only protected against UVB, and it wasn't until the 1990s that UVA was recognized as a cause of cancer. Many broad-spectrum sunscreens are available today. Use them, and don't forget the rims of your ears.

also find water- and sweat-resistant sun screens in stick form, such as Watermans Applied Science Face Stick Sunscreen. Sunscreen can be very irritating to the eyes, so avoid applying it above your eyes if it isn't sweat-proof.

SEXUAL DYSFUNCTION

The topic of bicycle saddles and erectile dysfunction (ED) has become controversial. In 1997, *Bicycling* magazine created a stir when it published an article citing an unpublished study by Irwin Goldstein, a nationally prominent urologist. Goldstein claimed that the pressure of the bicycle saddle on the main artery of the penis could eventually flatten or block it, causing restricted blood flow and ED. "There are two kinds of cyclists," he was quoted as saying, "those who are impotent, and those who will be."

An American television program, *20/20*, took up the baton and ran with the story. Soon, every cycling rag was issuing warnings about impotence. Goldstein's study was never subjected to peer review or replicated by other scientists. Many experts, including urologists, have expressed serious doubts as to its validity.

Most of the information concerning cycling and impotence is anecdotal in nature. Male cyclists often report numbness after many hours in the saddle, but this usually goes away after the ride has ended. Changing your saddle, position, or riding style will usually correct the problem. If you experience saddle discomfort or numbness, make sure your bicycle has been adjusted to fit you correctly, including the tilt of the saddle. Upward tilt places additional pressure in spots that are uncomfortable for men. A level saddle was considered preferable for comfort at one time; however, I have seldom found this to be the case with modern bikes and saddles. Greater comfort and performance can be obtained by tilting the saddle down slightly, ideally between 1.5 and 2.5 degrees. If you are still uncomfortable, try a different saddle with a cutout or soft padding in the appropriate places.

The best way to deal with injuries is to do everything you can to prevent them from occurring in the first place. Regular stretching, strength training, a good bike fit, and sufficient rest between workouts will help you avoid an injury. If you do experience an injury, treat it appropriately and allow sufficient time for it to heal. Finding the right balance of training and rest is essential for injury-free cycling and for enjoyment of the sport for life.

Glossary

abductors—The hip muscles that originate at the pubis and insert on the inside of the femur surface.

adductors—The three gluteal muscles and the tensor fasciae latae.

active recovery—Recovery while exercising at a less intense level.

aero—Aerodynamic.

aerobars—Handlebar extension that rests the hands close together over the front hub for an aerodynamic tuck.

aerobic—Exercise at an intensity that allows the body's need for oxygen to be continually met. This intensity can be maintained for long periods.

anaerobic—Exercise above the intensity at which the body's need for oxygen can be met. This intensity can be sustained for brief periods only.

anaerobic threshold (AT)—The transition between aerobic and anaerobic levels of exertion. Effective training increases AT by teaching the muscles to use oxygen more efficiently so that less lactic acid is produced. Also known as *lactate threshold*.

ancillary muscles—Muscles that are subordinate to the major muscles.

ANSI—A bicycle helmet standard set by the American National Standards Institute.

antioxidants—Compounds that react with free radicals to terminate the chain reactions they initiate.

apex—The sharpest part of the turn where the transition from entering to exiting takes place.

attack—A sudden acceleration to break away from other riders.

bike fitting—Adjusting the bike to fit the rider in a manner that will maximize power output and minimize stress to the body.

bike sizing—Matching the rider with a bike of a size that is most appropriate for the body dimensions of the rider.

blood lactate—The lactic acid salt that is produced as lactic acid diffuses from the muscle into the bloodstream.

bone mineral density (BMD)—The concentration of minerals, such as calcium, in the bones.

bonk—A state of severe exhaustion caused by the depletion of glycogen stores in the liver and muscles, which has been brought about by failure to eat and drink sufficiently.

bottom bracket—The part of the frame where the crankset is installed, including axle, cups, and bearings of the traditional crankset, or the cartridge of sealed-bearing cranksets.

brake calipers—The levers on the handlebars that pull the brake cable, thus activating the brakes.

brake levers—Mechanisms attached to the handlebars that control both the front-wheel and rear-wheel brakes on a bicycle with more than one gear.

brake pads—Rubber pads attached to the brake arms, which clamp the rim during braking.

breakaway—The leading rider or group of riders who have broken away from the peloton; a second rider or group of riders between the breakaway and the peloton is called the chase group.

brakehoods—Rubber covering of the brake calipers; hence "riding on the hoods" is riding with hands resting on the brakehoods.

brevet—Unsupported ultradistance rides that range in distance from 200 to 1,500 kilometers. Also known as *randonnées*.

bridging a gap—Going off the front of the peloton and making contact with a breakaway up the road.

cadence—Pedal revolutions per minute (rpm).

cantilever—Most common type of brake found on mountain bikes today. It is named for the two cantilever arms that pivot on the forks (front) or seat stays (rear).

carotenoids—Organic pigments that occur naturally in plants, algae, and some bacteria and fungi.

cassette—The set of gear cogs on the rear hub; also *freewheel,* or the vintage terms *cluster* or *block.*

chain—The flexible metal link between the rear wheel and the front chain ring. It transmits the power from the pedals to the rear wheel.

chain ring—A sprocket on the crankset; also a *ring,* such as big ring or small ring.

chain rings—The front gear wheels that drive the chain. Bicycles have one to three chain rings.

chain stay—Small tube running from the bottom bracket back to rear dropouts.

chain suck—Condition in which the bike chain gets jammed between the frame and the chain rings, or when the chain ring is so worn that it holds on to the chain and lifts it up to meet the incoming part of the chain.

chain tool—A tool designed to break the chain by extruding the pin from one of the links.

chamois—A soft, absorbent, slightly padded liner of the crotch of the cycling short, designed to be worn next to the skin.

chasers—A group of riders ahead of a peloton trying to catch a breakaway.

chondromalacia patellae—Painful condition that occurs when the cartilage that lines the patella (kneecap) becomes irritated.

circuit—A course that is ridden two or more times in a race.

cleat—A metal or plastic fitting on the sole of a cycling shoe that clips into the pedal.

clincher—Tire and tube are separate, and the tire expands under pressure to grip the sides of the rim like a car tire.

clipless pedals—Pedals designed for use with cleated shoes. The foot is secured to the pedal by attaching the cleat into the clipless pedal.

closed circuit—A racecourse that is completely closed to traffic. Closed circuits are most often used in criteriums or road races that use a relatively short lap (2 to 5 miles).

cockpit—The frontal region of the bicycle dealing with the extension of the rider on the machine.

cog—A sprocket on the rear wheel's cassette or freewheel.

core muscles—Muscles in the pelvic floor, abdomen (transversus abdominis, multifidus, obliques, diaphragm, and rectus abdominis), and back (erector spinae and longissimus thoracis) are the major groups, and minor core muscles are the latissimus dorsi, gluteus maximus, and trapezius.

crankset—A pair of crank arms, generally available in multiple lengths to better accommodate the dimensions of the rider.

criterium—A circuit race of multiple laps on a course that is about 1 mile or less.

cycling gloves—A glove, with or without fingers, with padding on the palm for comfort on the bars and protection from crashes.

cyclo-cross—A fall or winter race contested on a mostly off-pavement course with obstacles that force riders to dismount.

cyclometer—A device with a sensor that measures current speed, maximum speed, average speed, mileage, trip distance, and total distance. Some models also measure elevation change and include a clock and timer.

derailleur (front and rear)—Mechanism that moves the chain from one gear wheel to another. The front derailleur moves the chain on two or three chain rings. The rear derailleur moves the chain among as many as 10 cogs.

derailleur adjustment—A plastic or metal barrel where the shift cable enters the rear derailleur. Turning left or right adjusts where the derailleur hangs relative to the cogs on the freewheel. The front derailleur is usually adjusted by changing the cable attachment. Setscrews on front and rear derailleurs determine the full range of movement.

downshift—To shift to a lower gear (larger cog on the rear, smaller chain ring on the front).

downstroke—When the rider is pushing down on the pedal.

downtube—The tube extending from the bottom of the headset down to the bottom bracket.

drafting—Riding closely behind another rider in the slipstream (a pocket of moving air created by the rider in the front) decreases wind resistance. This enables the second rider to maintain speed with less effort. A drafting rider can save as much as 25 percent of effort and be more rested at the finish of the race.

drivetrain—Components directly involved in making the wheel turn: chain, crankset, and cassette.

drop—To outpace another rider and leave him or her behind.

dropout—An open-ended fixture at the fork ends and at the convergence of the seat and chain stays, which receive the axles of the wheels.

drops—Lower parts of a turned-down handlebar; also called the *hooks*.

echelon—A form of pace line used in a crosswind. Riders line up offset to the rider in front so the pace line stretches across the road at an angle.

endo—Short for *end over end*. The maneuver of flying unexpectedly over the handlebars, thus being forcibly ejected from the bike. Also known as a *Superman*.

EPO—Erythropoietin, the hormone that controls the production of red blood cells.

ergometer—A stationary bicycle-like device with adjustable resistance used in physiological testing or indoor training.

external hip rotators—Six muscles, including the piriformis, that fan out from the femur across the pelvis; when contracted, they rotate the femur outward and stabilize it in the hip joint.

feed zone—Designated areas on a racecourse where riders can be handed food and drinks. It is customary to feed from the right because most riders are right handed.

fiber, dietary—Indigestible soluble and insoluble plant material.

field sprint—The sprint for the finish line by the main group of riders.

fixed gear—A direct-drive power train using one chain ring and one rear cog with no freewheel mechanism. Used on track bikes, which have no derailleurs and no brakes and decrease speed with back pressure on the pedals. Also used on rollers or on road training bikes to improve pedaling technique.

flexibility—The range of motion of joints and muscles. Range of motion can be increased by stretching regularly.

flexion—The act of moving a limb so that the angle of the joint decreases; opposite of extension.

frame—The bike's chassis. Frames are made from a variety of materials, including steel, aluminum, titanium, and carbon fiber.

free radical—A highly reactive compound or an individual atom having at least one unpaired electron, which initiates a chain reaction that can damage important cell components, such as cell membranes or DNA.

freewheel—The cluster of gear wheels attached to the rear wheel, which provides a variety of gears.

front fork—Component of a bike frame that runs through the head tube forking around and over the front wheel to the front axle.

functional threshold power—Lactate threshold expressed in terms of power output.

gapped—When a rider falls back out of the draft of the rider in front, usually due to a sudden increase in speed by the rider in front, or to fatigue (see *drop*).

gear—Toothed wheel (sometimes called ring) that drives the chain.

gearshift lever—Lever used to switch gears by activating the front and rear derailleurs.

glutes—Muscle group. The gluteus maximus is the largest gluteal muscle, and it inserts at the gluteal tuberosity of the femur and the iliotibial band. The other two glutes are the gluteus medius and the gluteus minimus.

grupo—Includes crankset, brakes, calipers, and front and rear derailleurs.

hammer—To ride hard in big gears.

handlebars—The bicycle's steering apparatus.

handlebar tape—Tape used to cover the handlebars; usually made out of plastic, cork, or cloth. Some have foam padding.

headset—The bearing apparatus at the top and bottom of the head tube into which the stem and fork are fixed; should be adjusted snugly so there is no play, but not so tight that it binds.

headtube—Short vertical tube at the front of the frame.

heart-rate monitor—A wrist-mounted device that measures the heart rate through a chest sensor that is held in place by a strap during exercise.

helmet—Worn on the head to protect against head injury. Helmets should meet the standards of the American National Standards Institute (ANSI Z 90.4).

hill repeats—A series of aggressive hill climbs broken up by brief rest periods (descents) that increase cycling-specific leg strength.

hybrid bicycle—A bicycle that combines the features of a road bike and a mountain bike and is usually used for commuting and general transportation.

hypoxia—The limited availability of oxygen to parts or all of the body.

iliotibial band (IT band)—A tough, fibrous band of connective tissue that runs from the outside of the pelvis over the hip and knee, and inserts just below the knee. It is important for knee stabilization.

indoor trainer—Used for indoor training or for warming up before a race. A bicycle is attached to the indoor trainer unit by removing either the front or the rear wheel. The indoor trainer is a good training tool since the athlete can use his or her own bicycle.

interval training—A training method that alternates periods of hard effort with periods of rest.

jam—A period of hard, fast riding.

jump—A hard acceleration out of the saddle.

KOPS alignment—Knee over pedal spindle alignment, a rule commonly used as a starting point for adjusting the fore-and-aft position of the saddle.

lactate threshold—See *anaerobic threshold*.

lead-out—When one rider leads another to the line in his slipstream so the other can slingshot around the first rider for the final meters of the sprint. In any pack sprint, the first rider to go for the line is considered to be giving the lead-out.

ligament—A band of tough, fibrous connective tissue that connects one bone to cartilage or another bone.

kinesiology—The anatomy, physiology, and mechanics of bodily motion.

mass start—Any race event in which all contestants leave the starting line at the same time.

minuteman—The rider in front of another rider in the starting order of a time trial, so called because most time trials use a one-minute interval between starters, but correctly used no matter what the actual interval might be.

motor pace—To ride behind a motorcycle or other vehicle; usually done for speed work in training, but there are some motor-paced races on the track and on the road.

MTB—The activity of mountain biking, or a mountain bike itself.

muscle memory—When muscles repeatedly perform the same series of activities, physiological changes occur that improve the accuracy of the motion. This is also known as *neuromuscular facilitation.*

NORBA—National Off-Road Bicycling Association. As part of USAC, they organize most of the larger mountain bike races.

obliques—Two sets of core muscles (internal and external) located on the sides of the upper body. They are responsible for side-to-side and twisting motions.

off the back—When a rider fails to maintain contact with the main group.

osteoarthritis—The most common form of arthritis, which is pain and inflammation of the synovial joints due to erosion of the cartilage over time.

osteopenia—Lower-than-normal bone mineral density but not severe enough to be called osteoporosis.

osteoporosis—Low bone mineral density and an interruption in the microstructure of the bone, increasing the risk for fractures.

overgearing—Using too big a gear for the terrain or for one's conditioning.

overtraining—Condition when rider trains too much too soon, which leads to fatigue, injury, or burnout.

oxygen debt—The amount of oxygen that must be consumed to pay back the deficit incurred by anaerobic work.

pace line—A line of riders in which each lead rider pulls off at regular intervals, drops back to the last position, and begins to rotate through to the front of the line again. May be ridden with riders pulling off the front as soon as they are clear of the previous rider, thus creating a second line of riders dropping back to the rear position. May also be ridden as a double pace line in which the pair of riders at the front pull off simultaneously to the left and to the right.

parasympathetic nervous system—The part of the autonomic nervous system that acts in opposition to the sympathetic nervous system. For example, fear induces an increase in heart rate and respirations (fright-or-flight mode); the parasympathetic system works to slow the heart rate and calm the breathing.

peak—A relatively short time during which maximum performance is achieved.

pedals—The foot levers on the ends of the cranks that turn the chain rings.

peloton—The main group of riders in a race.

periodization—The division of training into progressive phases that allows the athlete to peak at a certain time and avoid overtraining and subsequent injury during the process.

phytoestrogens—Phytochemicals that are similar in chemical structure to estrogen and can act as mimics.

phytonutrients (or phytochemicals)—Nutrients that are obtained from plant sources.

picking a line—Planning the path of the bike by anticipating an approaching turn.

pinch flat—Internal puncture caused by rim pinching the tube when the wheel hits a hard object.

plant sterols—Steroid alcohols that occur naturally in plants and are thought to reduce cholesterol levels, reducing the risk for heart disease.

power meter—A device that usually measures torque with a strain gauge and uses this value along with angular velocity to calculate the power output.

Presta valve—Narrow valve stem with a small metal screw-down cap; common on light racing tires (see *Schrader valve*).

prime—Prize given to the leader of particular laps during a criterium or to the first rider to arrive at a designated line in a road race. Pronounced "preem."

pronation—When involving the foot, the sole tends to turn inward, that is, the weight of the individual is placed on the inside portion of the sole.

psi—Abbreviation of pounds per square inch; unit of measure for tire inflation.

pull—A turn taken on the front of a pace line; a breakaway of the peloton.

pull off—To move to the side after taking a pull.

Q-angle—Measurement of the angle formed by the intersection of a vertical line through the kneecap and a line from the hip through the kneecap.

quick-release—An over-top lever system attached for easy removal of wheels and adjustment of seat height.

randonneurs—Cyclists who ride in randonnées (see *brevets*).

recumbent—A bicycle on which the rider is in a reclining position.

resistance trainer—A stationary training device into which a bike is clamped.

rim—The outside section of a wheel around which the tube is inflated. Most rims are made of steel or aluminum. The tire covers the tube and holds it to the rim.

road race—Event that takes place on public roads (some have mass starts in which all the racers start at the same time from the same location). They can be point-to-point races or loops of 1 to 25 miles (40 km) in length.

road rash—Skin abrasion resulting from a crash, the most common cycling injury.

rollers—An indoor training device composed of three rollers (about 3 to 12 inches in diameter depending on the type of rollers) set parallel in a rectangular rack that rests on a flat surface.

saddle—The bicycle's seat.

saddle sores—Skin problem in the crotch that develops from chafing or excessive pressure caused by pedaling.

Schrader valve—Inner-tube valve like those found on car tires.

seat position—Height of seat from center of bottom bracket; fore-and-aft positioning of seat over bottom bracket; up-and-down tilt of seat.

seat stay—Small frame tubes descending from behind the seat to the rear dropouts.

seat tube—Frame tube running from the seat down to the bottom bracket.

sewup tire—A tire that is sewn together around its inner tube and glued onto a slightly concave rim. Also called a *tubular*.

shift lever—Modern shift levers are built into the brake calipers; before that, shift levers were placed near the top of the downtube.

single track—Trail just wide enough for one person, horse, or bike (the mountain biker's holy grail).

sit on a wheel—To ride in someone's draft.

skewer—The cam lever and spindle that clamps the hub of the wheel into the frame.

slipstream—Pocket of protected air behind a moving rider.

spin—Pedal at a high cadence.

spoke—The thin metal support rods that make up the inside of a wheel and keep the wheel round (or true).

spoke wrench—A wrench with a slot designed to fit the top of a spoke.

sprocket—General term for chain ring or cog.

stationary bicycle—Used for indoor training. The unit provides various levels of resistance.

steady state—Exercise performed at a level low enough to be maintained for prolonged periods. This type of exercise is mainly aerobic, which means that the amount of oxygen taken in to burn food satisfies energy requirements, so there is no oxygen deficit during exercise and no oxygen debt after the exercise.

stem—The bar that extends from the top of the headset to the handlebar.

supination—When involving the foot, the tendency for the sole of the foot to turn outward, that is, the weight of the individual is placed mostly on the outside portion of the soles.

synovial fluid—The pale, yellow, viscous liquid that acts as a medium for transporting nutrients, such as glucose, to the articular cartilage and facilitates motion by lubricating the joints.

take a flyer—To go very early in a sprint.

taper—To cut back mileage up to three weeks (depending on race distance) before a big race. Tapering helps muscles rest so that they are ready for peak performance on race day.

tempo—Fast riding at a brisk cadence.

tendon—A band of tough, fibrous connective tissue that attaches a muscle to a bone.

thread cut—When a puncture has cut one or more threads of the tire casing. (In that case, throw the tire away.)

time trial (TT)—Pitting individual riders against the clock with the goal of covering the course distance in the shortest time. The course is usually straight out for the 500-meter to 1-kilometer distances, and out and back for the 5-kilometer through 40-kilometer time trial.

tire—Rubber material that protects the tube. Tires come in a variety of sizes, depending on the size of the rim, and they come with various treads, depending on the terrain the bicycle is ridden on. Mountain bike tires are usually knobby; road-racing tires have a mixed or smooth tread.

toe clip—Toe piece attached to a pedal, which holds the shoe on the pedal.

top tube—The frame tube running from the seat to the top of the headset.

tubes—Rubber material that holds the air that keeps the tires inflated.

turn-around—The point where riders reverse direction on an out-and-back time-trial course.

twin track—Fire road that is like two parallel trails.

UCI—Union Cycliste Internationale, the international governing body of bicycle racing.

upshift—Shift to a higher gear, smaller cog, or larger chain ring.

USAC—acronym for USA Cycling, the governing body of professional and amateur bicycle racing in the United States.

velodrome—A banked track for bicycle racing.

$\dot{V}O_2$max—The maximum amount of oxygen that a person can extract from the atmosphere and then transport and use in the body's tissues.

Bibliography

CHAPTER 1

Harrop, JoAnne Klimovich. "Wheel Life – The National Cycling Festival shows the accelerating growth of the sport." http://www.masters-athlete.com/public/199.cfm.

Hunter, Allen and Andrew Coggan. *Training and Racing with a Power Meter*. Velo Press. 2005.

Kingsford, Rachel. "Bush's Mountain Biking Hobby." *Blue Ribbon Magazine*. June 2005. http://www.sharetrails.org/magazine/article.php?id=618

Moritz, W. "Survey of North American Bicycle Commuters: Design and Aggregate Results." *Transportation Research Record: Journal of the Transportation Research Board*. 1578, 101, 1997. http://pubsindex.trb.org/view.aspx?id=578182

National Association of Sporting Goods Retailers PDF file, 2007. http://www.nsga.org/files/public/2007rankedbytotal.080423.pdf

National Association of Sporting Goods Retailers, Survey, 2003.

Penseyres, Pete, Interview.

Pucher, J. and J. Renne. "Socioeconomics of Urban Travel: Evidence from the 2001 NHTS Transportation Quarterly." 2003. 57, 49-77. http://policy.rutgers.edu/faculty/pucher/TQPuchRenne.pdf

RAAM.com.

Royal, D. and D. Miller-Steiger. "National Survey of Bicyclist and Pedestrian Attitudes and Behavior." *National Highway Traffic Safety Administration*. 2008. http://www.nhtsa.dot.gov/portal/site/nhtsa/template.MAXIMIZE/menuitem.3d62007aac5298598fcb6010dba046a0/?javax.portlet.tpst=4670b93a0b088a006bc1d6b760008a0c_ws_MX&javax.portlet.prp_4670b93a0b088a006bc1d6b760008a0c_viewID=detail_view&itemID=545355f9ee1cb110VgnVCM1000002fd17898RCRD&overrideViewName=Article

Skufca, L. "Is the cost of gas leading Americans to use alternative transportation?" 2008. http://www.aarp.org/research/ppi/

Velo News. "Bike racing is growing in the U.S., USAC says." Posted December 8, 2008. http://velonews.competitor.com/?p=85769

CHAPTER 2

My Food Diary.com. "Exercise and Bone Density." 2010. http://www.myfooddiary.com/resources/ask_the_expert/exercise_bone_density.asp

Newswise.com. "Are Cyclists Pedaling Towards Osteoporosis?" 2010. http://www.newswise.com/articles/view/549615

Quinn, Elizabeth. "Advice for Older Athletes: Maintaining Fitness with Age." November, 2007. http://sportsmedicine.about.com/od/olderathletes/a/082404.htm

WebMD.com. "Bone Mineral Density." Healthwise, Inc. 2008. http://www.webmd.com/osteoporosis/bone-mineral-density

Wilks, D.C., S.F. Gilliver, and J. Rittweger. March 2009. Forearm and Tibial Bone Measures of Distance—and Sprint-Trained Master Cyclists. *Medicine & Science in Sports & Exercise,* 41(3): 566-573.

CHAPTER 3

Wallack, Roy M. and Bill Katovsky. *Bike for Life.* Marlowe and Company: New York, New York. 2005.

CHAPTER 4

Howard, John and Steve Tarpinian. "Stretching, Flexibility, and Speed." *Bicycle Guide.* October 1994.

"Performance Cycling Conditioning." *The Official Publication of the USA Cycling Coaching Association.* 8(3), 2002.

CHAPTER 5

Bike Cult.com. "Bicycle Roller Racing Machine." Bike Works: New York, New York. January, 2008. http://www.bikecult.com/works/rollers.html

Bike Cult.com. "Bicycle Tracks and Velodromes." July 2005. http://www.bikecult.com/bikecultbook/sports_velodromes.html

Bjorn, There. "Rolling the Night Away." Rapha.cc. February 2007. http://www.rapha.cc/index.php?page=122

Cycling Forums.com. "Cycling Acronyms Explained." February 2007. http://www.cycling-forums.com/cycling-training/386984-cycling-acronyms-ftp-vo2max-etc.html

Epic Idiot.com. "Indoor Bicycle Trainers: Beyond the Boredom." January, 2006. http://www.epicidiot.com/sports/indoor_training.htm

Hunter, Allen and Andrew Coggan. *Training and Racing with a Power Meter.* Velo Press. 2005.

Kreitler.com. "Kreitler Roller Accessories." December 2006. http://www.kreitler.com/product.php?section=product&item=accessories

Kreitler.com. "Which Kreitler Roller Model's Right for Me?" December 2006. http://www.kreitler.com/product.php?section=product&item=which_model

Racer Mate.com. "Computrainer." http://www.racermateinc.com/computrainer.asp

Road Bike Review.com. "Elite Parabolic Rollers, A Review." http://www.roadbikereview.com/cat/training/trainers/elite/PRD_331252_1663crx.aspx

Rocking Rollers.com. "Rocking Rollers." http://rockingrollers.com/pages/7/index.htm

Rollapaluza.com. "The History of Roller Racing." http://www.rollapaluza.com/?page_id=8

True Trainer.com. "Premium Bicycle Rollers." February 2008. http://www.trutrainer.com/products_rollers.shtml

Wikipedia.org. "Keith-Albee-Orpheum." http://en.wikipedia.org/wiki/Keith-Albee-Orpheum

CHAPTER 7

American Express Publications Corporation. "The 8 Health Benefits of Drinking Wine, Food and Wine." October 2007. http://www.foodandwine.com/articles/8-health-benefits-of-drinking-wine

Berry, Lynn. "Why We Need Action on Soil Depletion." Natural News.com. October 2008. http://www.naturalnews.com/024581_minerals_health_food.html

Carter, J. Stein. *Amino Acids and Proteins*. November 2004. http://biology.clc.uc.edu/courses/bio104/protein.htm

Christianson, Alan. *10 for the Road: Essential Nutrients for Endurance Athletes*. Penton Media, Inc. May 1999. http://www.newhope.com/nutritionsciencenews/NSN_backs/May_99/10for_road.cfm

EveryNutrient.com. "Health Benefits of Onions." 2006. http://www.everynutrient.com/healthbenefitsofonions.html

Food Democracy. "Chew on This – U.S. Soda Consumption." November 2007. http://food-democracy.wordpress.com/2007/11/09/chew-on-this-us-soda-consumption/

Fruit Desire.com. "Fruits for Athletes: Understanding Nutrition for Strength and Energy Without Chemical Drinks and Artificial Supplements." http://www.fruitdesire.com/fruits_for_athletes.html

Goff, H. Douglas. "Dairy Products: Overview and Fluid Milk Products." *University of Guelph, Dairy Science and Technology Education Series*. 2009. http://www.foodsci.uoguelph.ca/dairyedu/fluid.html

Hull, Janet Starr. *Alternative Health and Nutrition: Healthy Fats – The Benefits of Plant Sterols*. September 2007. http://www.janethull.com/newsletter/0907/healthy_fats_the_benefits_of_plant_sterols

Jackson Siegelbaum Gastroenterology. "High Fiber Diet." 2008. http://www.gicare.com/diets/high-fiber-diets.aspx

Larson, Enett. "Eating to Exercise and Compete." *The Vegetarian Resource Group*. August, 2006. http://www.vrg.org/nutshell/athletes.htm

Lehr, Lisa. "Wine and Beer Are Good For Us? Yes!" 2005. http://www.theworldwidewine.com/Wine_articles/Wine_and_health/wbga.php

Levin, Rachel. "The Healthy Benefits of Beer." *The Food Paper*. 2006. http://www.thefood-paper.com/features/health/beer.html

Michelle, C. "Tannins Found in Cranberries Act as Antibacterial Agents." *Health and Wellness*. Associated Content.com. November 2007. http://www.associatedcontent.com/article/448176/tannins_found_in_cranberries_act_as.html?cat=5

Michalek, Joel E., et al. "Effects of the AlgaeCal Bone-Health Program on Bone Mineral Density (BMD)." April, 2008. http://www.algaecal.com/trace-minerals.html

Mother Nature, Inc. *Phytonutrients*. 1995-2009. http://www.mothernature.com/Library/Bookshelf/Books/23/54.cfm

Penton Media, Inc. "Mintel: Carbonated Soft Drink Consumption Loses Fizz." April 2009. http://supermarketnews.com/news/mintel_carbonated_0402/

Reuters.com. "Learn About the Consumer's Hot and Soft Drink Preferences: New Trends and Perspectives." January, 2008. http://www.reuters.com/article/pressRelease/idUS28031+20-Jan-2008+BW20080120

Ryan, Monique. "The Feedzone with Monique Ryan: Nutrition planning for an important race." Velo News.com. June, 2007. http://velonews.com/article/12445

Sears, William. "Eggs." *Family Nutrition.* 2006. http://www.askdrsears.com/html/4/T041100.asp

Sears, William. "Fabulous Fruits." *Family Nutrition.* 2006. http://www.askdrsears.com/html/4/T042600.asp#T042603

Sport Quest Direct.com. "Protein Supplementation." http://www.nvo.com/sportquestdir/proteinsupplementation/#calcium

USDA. "My Pyramid.gov: Steps to a Healthier You." September 2009. http://www.mypyramid.gov/pyramid/index.html

Weed, Duane. "Natural Health School Free Herbalist Training Program, Lesson 18: pH Balance." http://www.naturalhealthschool.com/acid-alkaline.html

Welloria.com. "Sodas: Passion for Fizz." June 2006. http://www.welloria.com/Soft_Drinks/Carbonated_Soda_Pop_History_Diet_Nutrition_Health_p1.html

Wikipedia.org. "Adaptogen." June 2009. http://en.wikipedia.org/wiki/Adaptogen

Wikipedia.org. "Resveratrol." September 2009. http://en.wikipedia.org/wiki/Resveratrol

Wine Lovers Page.com. "The Numbers that the Label Won't Show You." http://www.wineloverspage.com/wines/nutrition.shtml

Women to Women.com. "Symptoms-Joint Pain and Stiffness." *Women to Women.* 2010. http://www.womentowomen.com/understandyourbody/symptoms/stiffnessjointpain.aspx,

World of Molecules.com. "Food Molecules: Lutein and Zeaxanthin." http://www.worldofmolecules.com/antioxidants/lutein_zeaxanthin.htm

CHAPTER 8

Bernardi, L., et.al. "Respiratory and Cardiovascular Adaptations to Progressive Hypoxia – Effect of Interval Hypoxic Training." *European Heart Journal.* 2001. 22: 879-886.

Quinn, Elizabeth. "Preventing Overtraining – When Less is More." About.com. http://sportsmedicine.about.com/cs/overtraining/a/aa062499a.htm.

Roels, B., et.al. "Effects of Hypoxic Interval Training on Cycling Performance." *Journal of Applied Physiology.* 2005. 98(1): 186-92. Epub. 2004 March 19.

Selye, Hans. "The Nature of Stress." Reprinted from *The Best of Basal Facts.* http://www.icnr.com/articles/thenatureofstress.html

CHAPTER 9

Bicycleforlife.org. "Bicycle for Life: RUSA Brevets." http://www.bicycleforlife.org/rusa/brevet.html.

Howard, John. "Training for Ultras: Flexibility First." *Ultra Cycling.* January/February 2002. 2(1).

CHAPTER 10

Arthritistoday.org. "What is Osteoarthritis?" *Arthritis Today*. March 2010. http://www.arthritistoday.org/conditions/osteoarthritis/all-about-oa/what-is-oa.php

Bernhardt, Gale. "Women-Only Cycling Issues Explained." Active.com. http://www.active.com/cycling/Articles/Women-Only_Cycling-Issues-Explained.htm.

Cancer Council Victoria. "Skin Cancers (non-melanoma)." December 2007. http://www.cancervic.org.au/about-cancer/cancer_types/skin_cancers_non_melanoma#skin_in_the_sun

Chain Reaction.com. "About the Bicycling Magazine and 20/20 News Story on, er…." September, 2007.

Cluett, Jonathan. "How to Heal a Broken Bone Quickly." *About.com Guide*. July 2009. http://orthopedics.about.com/od/castsfracturetreatments/ht/quickly.htm

Dermis.net. "What are the Main Functions of the Skin?" March 2010. http://skincancer.dermis.net/content/e01geninfo/e6/index_eng.html

McCorkell, Charlie. "Get Off That Bike if You Value Your Penis." Conference sponsored by the New York University School of Medicine. December, 2000. http://www.cars-suck.org/research/wilting.html

Quinn, Elizabeth. "Skin Abrasions and Road Rash Treatment." *About.com Guide*. August, 2007. http://sportsmedicine.about.com/cs/injuries/a/abrasions.htm

Veloist.com. "Geezer on a Bike." *The Veloist*. 2007. http://www.veloist.com/2007/10/sex-and-cycling-or-why-can-man-cream.html.

Veloist.com. "Sex and Cycling." *The Veloist*. 2007. http://www.veloist.com/2007/10/sex-and-cycling-or-why-can-man-cream.html.

Index

Note: The italicized *t* and *f* following page numbers refer to tables and figures, respectively.

About the Author

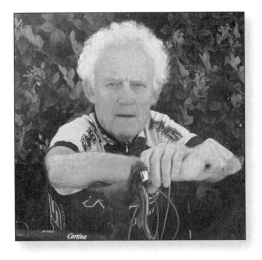

John Howard has a remarkable resumé as a professional cyclist, endurance athlete, and coach. He spent 10 years on the U.S. national cycling team and raced in three Olympic Games. In 1971, he won first place in the Pan-Am Games road race—America's only gold medal ever in that event. He has won other major road races, including the Tour de L'Estra, the Tour of Newfoundland, and the Tour of Baja. An American pioneer on the European racing circuit, he won a stage and finished third overall in the Tour of Ireland in 1973. John was a cofounder of the coast-to-coast Race Across America (RAAM) and finished second in the inaugural race. In 1987, he set the 24-hour cycling distance record of 539 miles (867 km). In 1989, he was inducted into the U.S. Cycling Hall of Fame.

Howard's achievements don't end with traditional bike racing. In 1985, he set the bicycle speed record of 152.2 mph (245 kph), riding behind a custom-built land rocket on the Bonneville Salt Flats. He won the Hawaii Ironman Triathlon in 1981. In 2000, he set the 24-hour canoeing record of 104.6 miles (168.4 km). He has been named a masters cycling national champion an unprecedented 18 times. He now runs one of cycling's best-regarded coaching clinics, the John Howard School of Champions. By his estimation, John has ridden more than 1/2 million miles during his career.

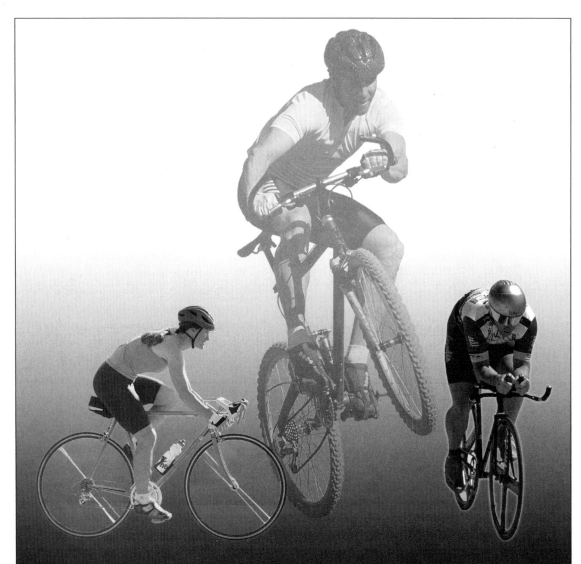

You'll find other outstanding cycling resources at

www.HumanKinetics.com/cycling

In the U.S. call 1-800-747-4457

Australia 08 8372 0999 • Canada 1-800-465-7301
Europe +44 (0) 113 255 5665 • New Zealand 0800 222 062

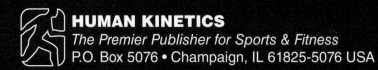

HUMAN KINETICS
The Premier Publisher for Sports & Fitness
P.O. Box 5076 • Champaign, IL 61825-5076 USA